D1097099

Clinical Foundations

NEUROMUSCULAR TECHNIQUES, SPORTS MASSAGE, AND MYOFASCIAL MASSAGE

Second Custom Edition for

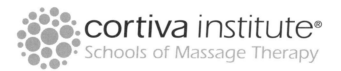
cortiva institute®
Schools of Massage Therapy

Learning Solutions

New York   Boston   San Francisco
London   Toronto   Sydney   Tokyo   Singapore   Madrid
Mexico City   Munich   Paris   Cape Town   Hong Kong   Montreal

Cover Art: PhotoDisc/Getty Images

Copyright © 2011 by Pearson Learning Solutions
All rights reserved.

This copyright covers material written expressly for this volume by the editor/s as well as the compilation itself. It does not cover the individual selections herein that first appeared elsewhere. Permission to reprint these has been obtained by Pearson Learning Solutions for this edition only. Further reproduction by any means, electronic or mechanical, including photocopying and recording, or by any information storage or retrieval system, must be arranged with the individual copyright holders noted.

All trademarks, service marks, registered trademarks, and registered service marks are the property of their respective owners and are used herein for identification purposes only.

Pearson Learning Solutions, 501 Boylston Street, Suite 900, Boston, MA 02116
A Pearson Education Company
www.pearsoned.com

Printed in the United States of America

1 2 3 4 5 6 7 8 9 10 V312 16 15 14 13 12 11

000200010270737810

SB/LP

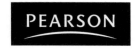

ISBN 10: 0-558-99806-2
ISBN 13: 978-0-558-99806-6

CONTENTS

Stretching

FLEXIBILITY

Flexibility is a major component of physical fitness. A balance of flexibility and strength is necessary to tone muscles so that the body moves efficiently and smoothly. Muscles, connective tissue, ligaments and tendons need to be supple and flexible enough to allow normal range of motion (ROM) around a joint. Restricted joint motion leads to aches, pain, joint disorders, and disability.

Massage therapy, and its benefits, directly influence an individual's ability to maintain or increase flexibility. Incorporating stretching techniques can greatly contribute to a client's ability to overcome deficits in flexibility and help optimize that individual's range of motion throughout the body.

Flexibility Defined

Flexibility: the degree of range of motion around a joint.

Optimal Flexibility: a balance of a joint's ability to perform the range of motion required of it and the body's ability to maintain the integrity of the joint.

The Physiology of Flexibility

Many factors are involved in determining an individual joint's flexibility or range of motion. To understand these factors, one must look to the anatomy of a joint and the physiology that determines a joint's ability to move in certain ways.

Factors That Limit Joint Range of Motion

1. The bony structure of the joint.

2. The ligamentous structure of the joint.

3. Musculo-tendinous structures around the joint.

Causes of Inflexibility

Aside from the normal limits to range of motion listed above, there are several common factors that lead to diminished or abnormal range of motion.

1. Muscle imbalance

2. Muscles in a state of partial contraction

3. Underuse

4. Overuse

5. Loss of tissue elasticity

6. Periods of rapid growth in height or weight.

Negative Effects of Inflexibility

Diminished flexibility can have many negative and potentially unhealthy effects for the individual.

1. Poor posture

2. Increased risk of injury

3. Poor muscular health

4. Energetically draining

5. Psychologically defeating

6. Restricts activities

7. Affects breathing and organ function

8. Inhibits circulation

Two Approaches To Improving Flexibility of a Muscle or Muscle Group Are:

1. Decrease the tension of, or on, the tight muscle(s) (stretching)

2. Increase the strength of the antagonistic muscle(s) (strengthening)

PASSIVE STRETCH

Stretching techniques have historically been used as a complement to the application of manual therapy techniques. Pehr Henrik Ling included stretching along with massage in his *Swedish Gymnastics*. Although there are varied and changing opinions about which stretching techniques are most effective and when, almost everyone agrees that some kind of stretching has a positive effect on mobility and performance.

Passive stretching can be an integral component of any massage session and it is often used in Sports Massage to help return tissues to their normal length after exercise. Stretching is often used to increase general flexibility and overall health. In addition to increasing range of motion, passive stretching can be a way of increasing a client's body awareness. Feeling the effects of a passive stretch during a massage can help motivate clients to maintain stretching as a self-care activity.

STRETCHING DEFINED

Stretching: Specific procedures designed and practiced to maintain or increase flexibility through physical elongation of tissues and/or retraining of the neuromuscular system.

TYPES OF STRETCHING

Ballistic Stretching

- With a bouncing or pulsing rhythmic motion.
- Dynamic, kinetic and fast stretching.
- High-force, short duration movements.

Ballistic stretching stimulates the muscle spindles which control the stretch reflexes. In doing so, the stretch of the muscle spindle actually causes reflex contraction, the opposite response that a stretch should provoke.

Static Stretching

- A controlled and slow stretch held at the point of resistance.
- Does not incorporate continuous movement.
- Reduces muscle tension.
- Less likely to impose potential injurious forces on the muscle.

Static stretching stimulates the Golgi Tendon Organ, causing relaxation of the muscle spindle and the entire muscle group.

METHODS OF STRETCHING

Passive Stretching

No active contraction is made by the individual being stretched. The motion is performed by another individual or outside force responsible for the stretch. The action should be slow and steady, using gentle movement to lengthen soft tissues. This is an example of static stretching. This lengthening will allow greater ROM of the affected joints.

Active Stretching

Motion and stretch through the contraction and relaxation of one's own muscles without outside aid. Active stretching can be ballistic or static. Active stretching during a massage treatment can be used to give a client more control over the stretch. Active stretching is also used for the purposes of the therapist or client's self-care.

Active Assisted Stretching

The individual performs active contraction of a muscle group until the limit of flexibility is reached. At this point the range of motion is completed by another person.

There are also stretching techniques that require a client's resistance. Examples of this include contract-relax and reciprocal inhibition. This will be discussed in the proprioceptive neuromuscular facilitation (PNF) section of this manual.

THE PHYSIOLOGY OF STRETCHING

Stretching, and the effectiveness of stretching, is dependent on the neuromuscular mechanism and the connective tissue interrelationship.

The central nervous system (CNS) and its activity determine the degree of tone and contraction or relaxation in a muscle.

In order for a muscle to stretch, the nervous system needs to inhibit contraction of that muscle's fibers. Stretching retrains the neuromuscular system and sets the stage for a return to muscle balance.

Hyper- or Hypotonicity

- Tone is a state of partial contraction that allows the muscle to stay in a state of readiness. Tone determines the normal resting length of the muscle, or in the case of pathology, creates hyper- or hypotonicity.

- One of the most significant elements in stretching is the state of the connective tissues.

- *The action of stretching places tension on fascial tissues around a joint.* Holding a stretch position allows time for fascia to warm and change to a more liquid consistency (thixotropy) and induces movement in a particular direction. Fascial tissues that are 'cold,' or in a more gel-like state, will restrict elongation and movement.

- Whether due to trauma, injury, immobilization, disease or postural strain, fascial elongation can be limited by two additional factors:

Shortened Fascial Tissues

- A common result of pathology is a shortening of fascia. Fascia tends to be drawn towards areas of injury or stress. Fascia drawn away from a joint can limit that joint's range of movement. In addition, the connective tissues that envelop each muscle fascicle, fiber and belly (epi-, peri- and endomysium), as well as the tendons, can become chronically shortened. These fascial tissues must be elongated for homeostasis to return to the area.

Fascial Adhesion

- The binding of fascial tissues of different layers inhibits free joint and muscular movement by restricting or limiting the distance they can be moved or stretched. These different layers must be able to glide freely over each other. They must have the ability to move freely.

- Beyond the influence of the nervous system on muscle tone, the muscle itself has a role in determining its ability to lengthen. Fibrils within the muscle fibers and within each muscle belly must individually and as a group be able to lengthen. *Stretching places tension on the muscle fibrils/fibers provoking them to elongate.* There is one factor within the muscle that might inhibit a positive response to stretching.

Muscular Binding or Adhesion

- A muscle may have an inability to elongate because of binding or adhesion within the muscle belly. Muscle tissues and their surrounding connective tissues, when subjected to stress (particularly when combined with immobilization), can adhere to themselves and create additional restriction. These fibers will be inhibited from exercising their full ability to contract or elongate and, therefore, will not be able to move freely. In order for a muscle to lengthen, the muscle fibers must be able to move freely.

- (Stretching stimulates the Golgi Tendon Organs and signals the nervous system to relax the muscle. No clear evidence that this occurs.)

SUMMARY

These important elements work together to allow or limit flexibility and the ability of the therapist or client to effectively perform stretching techniques. Specific massage techniques can be used to prepare the tissues and nervous system and increase the effectiveness of stretching techniques. Stretching techniques appeal to these factors to create elongation and increase range of motion.

To Summarize—Stretching

- Retrains the neuromuscular system.
- Elongates shortened and adhered connective tissues.
- Decreases binding in the muscle fibers.

STRETCHING AND THE STRETCH REFLEX

Protective Mechanisms for Stretching

When performing both active and passive stretching techniques, be mindful of proper positioning and biomechanics for yourself and your client. Executing stretching techniques in a careless and insensitive manner can cause injury and activate a protective reflex that will counteract the stretch you are imposing.

Muscle Spindle Organs, Golgi Tendon Organs and the Stretch Reflex

The organs responsible for these protective reflexes are the Muscle Spindle Cells and the Golgi Tendon Organs. Both organs work in concert to supply the central nervous system with information about the forces being generated in and around the muscle.

Muscle Spindle Cells are mechanoreceptors that are found in the muscle belly. They transduce (convert from one form of energy into another form of energy) information about changes in the length of a muscle (stretch) and the velocities at which those changes are taking place.

When the Muscle Spindle Cells' input to the CNS approaches threshold, a reflex is initiated that causes *contraction* or shortening in the muscle in which the Muscle Spindle Cell is housed. This response is called a **stretch or myotatic reflex.** This sudden contraction counters the stretching forces to prevent further elongation and potential injury to the tissues. The degree of the reflex or contraction is dependent upon the force and/or velocity of the stretch being applied. Activating a stretch reflex is, therefore, usually counter productive to a stretch because the muscle is contracting and actually getting shorter. For this reason, a "ballistic" or bouncing stretch is usually not recommended.

Golgi Tendon Organs are found in tendons, in the connective tissue within skeletal muscle, and around joints. They monitor the stretching force (tension) imposed upon these structures.

When the Golgi Tendon Organs' input to the CNS approaches threshold, a reflex is initiated that causes relaxation in the muscle in which they are housed. This response is called an inverse myotatic reflex. In stretching, it is these organs that counteract the muscle spindle's stretch reflex by immediately signaling the muscle to relax after the contraction.

Both of these receptors are considered to be proprioceptors because of the important roles they play in relaying information to the CNS about posture, movement, changes in equilibrium and external forces acting upon the body.

Regular stretching increases the muscle's ability to lengthen and increase the range of motion before activating muscle contraction by way of the stretch reflex.

BENEFITS OF STRETCHING

1. Increase/maintain ROM
2. Increase local circulation by freeing capillary restrictions
3. Increase muscle relaxation
4. Promote body awareness
5. Elongate fascia
6. Relieve muscle/joint stiffness
7. May help to decrease the risk of injury to musculo-tendinous unit
8. Improve sense of body integration coordination through freer movement
9. Decrease the pain-spasm-pain cycle
10. Maintain muscle balance—dominant vs. non-dominant/injury vs. non-injury
11. Psychological benefits
    - Kinesthetic awareness for the client
    - Feels good

Before Exercise

- Warms muscle tissue
- Increases elasticity

After Exercise

- Increases blood flow to fatigued areas
- Helps carry away metabolites (waste products of cellular metabolism)
- Decreases muscle soreness
- Restores over-contracted (tight) muscles to pre-exercise length.

CONTRAINDICATIONS TO STRETCHING

1. Inflammatory Conditions—especially in the joint
   a. Arthritis
      i. Osteo
      ii. Rheumatoid
      iii. Others
   b. Bursitis
2. Acute pain or any condition in which movement produces pain
3. Lax ligamenture—joints prone to dislocation, displacement or subluxation
4. Certain medications
   a. Injectable steroids
   b. Blood thinners
   c. Others
5. Pregnancy cautions
6. Abnormal joint structure
7. Surgical implants and appliances
8. Severe nerve root pain or radiating symptoms
9. Advanced diabetes
10. Bone diseases
11. Spinal or skeletal paralysis
12. Certain neuroses
13. Inability to 'let go'
14. Hypermobility
15. Recent injury
16. Scarring in connective tissue
17. Loss of muscle tissue

Muscle Length and Muscle Health

An additional caution involves chronically over-lengthened muscles. Muscles subject to over-lengthening tend to become weaker. Muscles in these conditions typically do not benefit from additional stretching and may lead to further pathology.

PASSIVE STRETCH

Performing a passive stretch can help increase the flexibility at a joint as well as the soft tissues surrounding the joint in order to lengthen the muscle fibers. In order to do this, the therapist needs to understand joint structure, muscle attachments and actions, proper positioning of the client and the therapist, and proper application of the stretch. The movement is applied in a specific direction to the limit of a particular joint.

GUIDELINES FOR PASSIVE STRETCHING

Warming Tissue/Self-Stretching
Precede stretching with a 5–10 minute aerobic warm-up to increase blood flow and oxygen to tissues (i.e., biking, jogging, brisk walking).

Therapist/Client Passive Stretching
Precede stretching with compression and movement to lubricate synovial capsules, bring blood into an area, create some release of fascial tissue and increase tissue receptivity.

General Guidelines
1. The muscles should be warmed through either exercise or massage prior to stretching.
2. Begin a stretch slowly.
3. Be specific—identify and isolate the muscle to be stretched.
   - Use visual, verbal and tactile clues for the client to identify where (and where not) to feel the stretch.
4. Use proper breathing—slow, rhythmical and natural.
   - Exhale as the body part engages in the stretch.
   - Inhale as the body part resumes the starting position.
5. Relax the area and muscle to be stretched so the fibers lengthen.
6. Hold a stretch for a minimum of 20 seconds but not to exceed 1–2 minutes.
7. Do not use bouncing or jerking movements which may injure connective tissues.
8. A stretch should be felt in the belly of the muscle and not in the joint.
9. Do not force a stretch beyond a comfortable zone. There should be no muscle pain.
10. In order for the stretch to be effective, correct body alignment of the client and proper body mechanics of the therapist are extremely important.
11. Listen to your own body. Adapt the stretch to 'fit' your own body structure or find stretches that suit your body.
12. Every individual varies in his/her flexibility and the ROM that may be achieved.

Modifying Stretches
Degrees of flexibility vary widely among individuals and even among different muscles and joints in a person's body. For those who are less flexible, try simpler stretch positions that isolate the stretch to a single muscle group (or fewer muscle groups) or change the relationship of the body to gravity.

Sample Script of A Stretching Procedure
"We are going to do passive stretch for the __hamstrings__."
"The __hamstrings__ are located on the __posterior thigh__." At the same time, show the client visually on yourself where they should feel the stretch. Touch the area on the client's body where the stretch should be felt.
"You should feel this stretch in the belly of the muscle, not at the __hip or knee joints__."
"Take a breath in and slowly exhale. Let me know when you begin to feel the stretch in the belly of the muscle."
"Continue breathing normally as I hold this stretch for about twenty seconds."

Gastrocnemius/Soleus (Pushing)

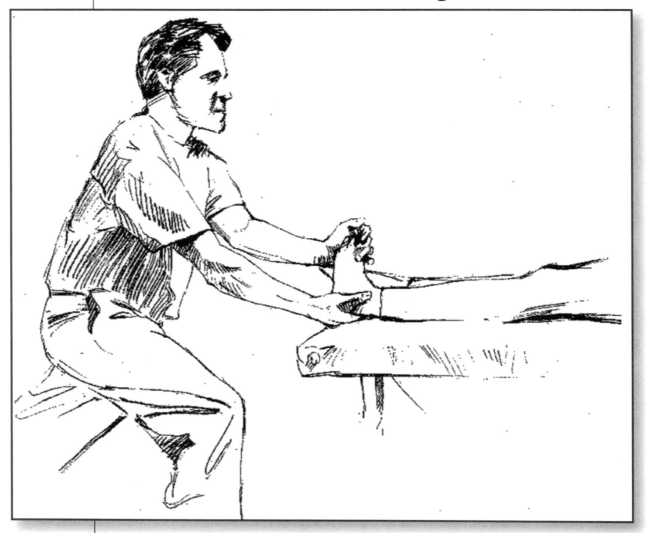

Client's Position

Supine and with the feet at the end of the table to assist the therapist in maintaining good body mechanics.

Passive Stretch Procedure

1. Stand in a foot-forward position or kneel in a lunge position at the foot of the table.

2. Stabilize the ankle with your outside hand supporting the lateral malleolus and your inside hand at the ball of the foot.

3. Dorsiflex the ankle toward the client's head.

Considerations

Many clients will feel resistance or no stretch in the calf area. If so:

a. Pull with your outside hand, thus stretching the Achilles tendon while simultaneously dorsiflexing the client's ankle.

b. Have the client sit upright.

Gastrocnemius/Soleus (Pulling)

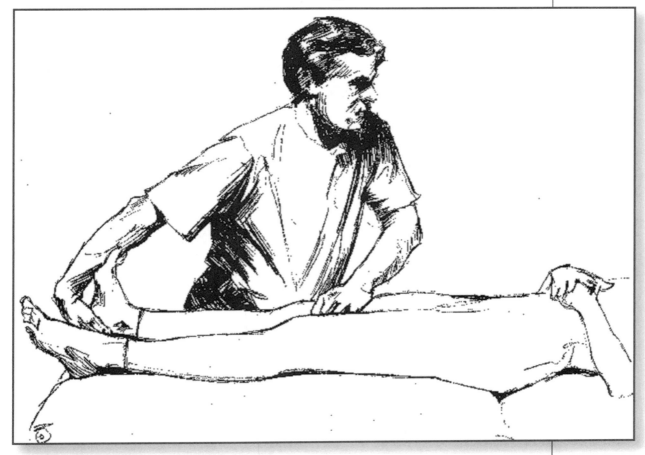

Client's Position

Supine with feet at the end of the table to assist the therapist in maintaining good body mechanics.

Passive Stretch Procedure

1. Stand at the side of the table in a lunge position facing the head of the table.

2. Stabilize the foot/ankle with your inside/inferior hand with the client's heel in your palm and the ball of the foot against your forearm. Stabilize the leg proximal to the knee joint with your outside/superior hand.

   Caution: Avoid hyperextension of the knee joint.

3. Dorsiflex the ankle toward the client's head using your weight and leverage from the lunge position.

Considerations

Many clients will feel resistance or no stretch in the calf area. If so:

a. Lean forward into a low lunge position. The client may be receiving more hip elevation than dorsiflexion of the ankle.

b. Have the client sit upright.

Some therapists' hands and forearms are short relative to the size of the client's foot, thus this technique may not be suitable.

Hamstrings (Straight Leg)

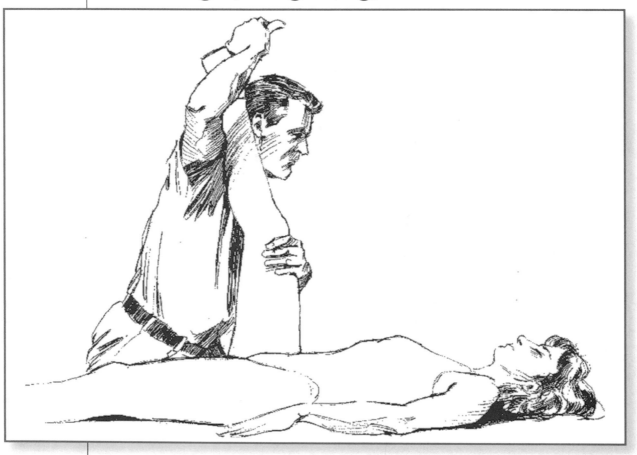

Client's Position

Supine at the edge of the table, to assist the therapist in maintaining proper body mechanics.

Passive Stretch Procedure

1. Stand in a lunge position facing the head of the table.

2. Stabilize the client's straight leg just proximal to the knee joint with your outside hand; the inside hand is placed behind the client's ankle or over the ball of the foot.

3. Flex the hip in an arc-like fashion toward the client's head.

Considerations

Many clients will feel restriction or a stretch behind the knee joint or in the calf before they feel a stretch in the hamstrings. If so, slightly flex the client's knee until restriction or a stretch is not felt in those areas, then proceed with hip flexion.

Adductor Group (Straight Leg)

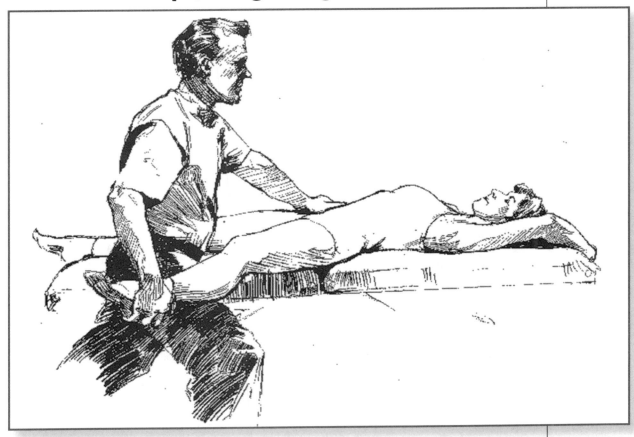

Client's Position

Supine and at the edge of the table to assist the therapist in maintaining proper body mechanics.

Passive Stretch Procedure

1. Face the head of the table. Stand in a lunge position between the client's leg and the table.

2. Stabilize the client's straight leg just distal to the ankle joint with your outside hand. Be sure the client's foot points toward the ceiling. Stabilize at the client's opposite anterior superior iliac spine (ASIS) with your inside hand.

3. Maintaining the leg at the horizontal level of the massage table, abduct the hip in an arc-like fashion outward from the table. Use your bodyweight, moving forward with the lunge to apply or enhance the stretch.

Considerations

Therapists with short arms relative to the client's legs may need to stabilize the straight leg just distal to the knee joint with the superior hand.

Be sure the client's foot points toward the ceiling while taking the leg through abduction. If the foot is turned toward the client's head, it rotates the femur and becomes more of a hamstring stretch than adductor stretch, creating an illusion of greater abduction range of motion.

Be sure the client's opposite ASIS, or upper leg, is stabilized. If it isn't, the client's pelvis and lower torso will rotate toward the leg that is stretching. This usually creates an illusion of greater range of motion and/or means the client will not realize a significant stretch in the adductor muscles.

Adductor Group (Figure 4)

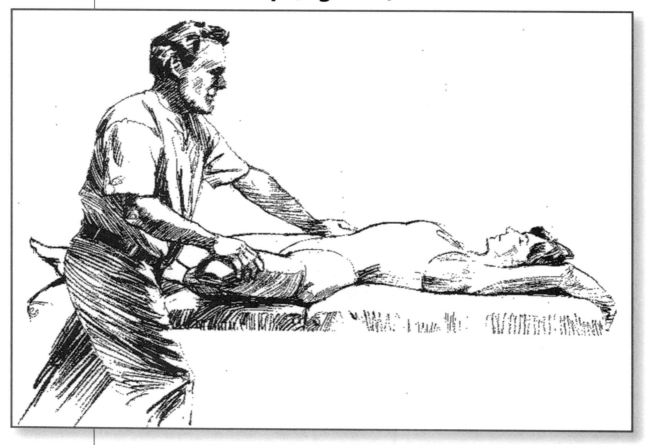

Client's Position

Supine and at the end of the table to assist the therapist in maintaining proper body mechanics. The client's knee is flexed, with the sole of the foot against the opposite knee joint; the hip is flexed, with the leg (knee) abducted.

Passive Stretch Procedure

1. Stand facing the head of the table.

2. Stabilize the client's leg at the medial aspect of the knee joint with your outside hand; stabilize the client's opposite anterior superior iliac spine (ASIS) with your inside hand.

3. Abduct the hip by pushing the client's knee toward the floor.

Considerations

Be sure the client's opposite ASIS, or upper leg, is stabilized. If it isn't, the client's pelvis and lower torso will rotate toward the leg that is stretching, creating an illusion of greater range of motion, which may mean the client will not realize a significant stretch in the adductor muscles.

Be sure the client's low back, sacrum and sacro-iliac joints are not being strained or subjected to any discomfort. To achieve a good safe stretch, try stabilizing the opposite ASIS by rolling the hip further away and then abducting.

The client's low back and hips always remain firmly in contact with the table to avoid any arching or straining of the client's back.

Quadriceps

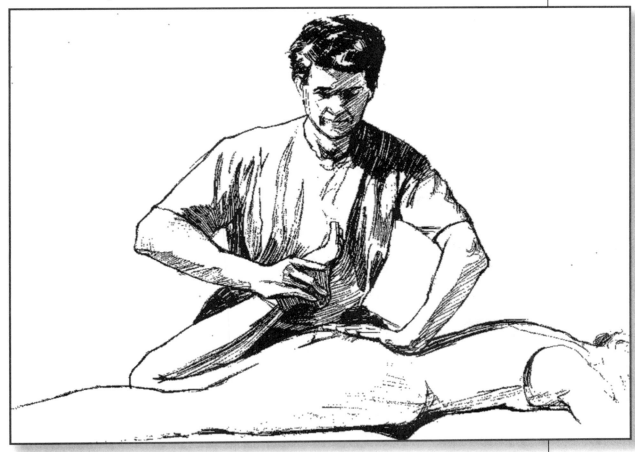

Client's Position
Prone; both ASISes stay in contact with the table throughout the stretch.

Passive Stretch Procedure
1. Stand in a lunge position facing the side of the table at a slight angle.
2. Stabilize the client's sacrum with your superior hand; stabilize the leg proximal to the ankle with your inferior hand. Be sure the leg is in a straight line with the body.
3. Flex the knee joint by bringing the foot toward the client's hip.

Considerations
Many clients will be flexible enough for the ankle to reach the hip without a stretch, or will not feel a stretch in the quadriceps area; if so:

a. Support the sacrum more and/or slightly decompress the sacrum toward the client's feet.
b. Be sure the leg being stretched is in a straight line with the body and is not abducted.
c. Have the client tighten his or her abdominal muscles as the stretch is applied (pelvic tilt).

Abductors—Tensor Fascia Latae/Gluteus Medius (1 of 2)

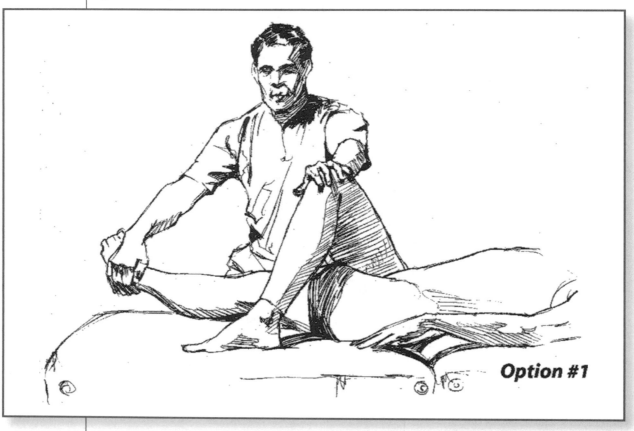

Option #1

Client's Position

Supine at the edge of the table to assist the therapist in maintaining proper body mechanics. The leg to be stretched is straight; the other leg is flexed at the hip and knee, with the foot placed on the table crossing the knee of the straight leg.

Passive Stretch Procedure

1. Stand on the same side of the table as the bent leg.

2. Stabilize the straight leg just distal to the ankle joint with your outside hand. Make sure the client's foot points toward the ceiling. Stabilize the client's other leg at the knee with your inside hand.

3. Adduct the hip in by moving the straight leg in an arc-like fashion toward your side of the table.

Considerations

Therapists with short arms relative to the client's legs may need to stabilize the straight leg just distal to the knee joint. The therapist then uses his or her own leg in a lunge position to support the weight of the client's leg. It may be helpful to ask the client to move toward the edge of the table or to lie on a diagonal.

To target the stretch for the gluteus medius muscle, flex the client's hip higher than the table and maintain the leg in a straight position while moving through adduction.

Be sure the client's pelvis is stabilized by stabilizing the knee of the uninvolved leg. If it isn't, the client's pelvis and lower torso will rotate toward the side where the leg is being stretched. This creates an illusion of greater range of motion and/or means the client will not experience a significant stretch in the abductor muscles.

The client may not feel a stretch in the intended muscle if his/her thighs are being compressed together, as that won't allow for full adduction. Try re-positioning the flexed leg so it is out of the way.

Abductors—Tensor Fascia Latae/Gluteus Medius (2 of 2)

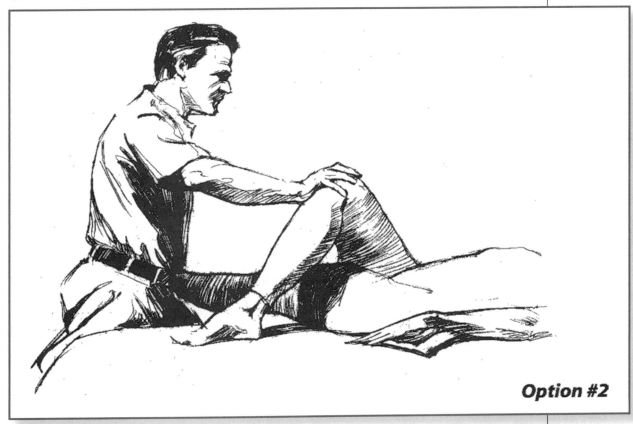

Option #2

Client's Position

Supine at the edge of the table to assist the therapist in maintaining proper body mechanics. The leg to be stretched is straight; the other leg is flexed at the hip and knee, with the foot placed on the table crossing the knee of the straight leg.

Passive Stretch Procedure

1. Face the head of the table. With the straight leg adducted, stand in a lunge between the client's leg and the table.

2. Stabilize the straight leg just proximal to the ankle joint with your outside hand; stabilize the client's other leg at the knee with your inside hand.

3. Maintaining the straight leg at the horizontal level of the table, adduct the hip in an arc-like fashion toward your side of the table.

Considerations

Therapists with short arms relative to the client's legs may need to stabilize the straight leg just distal to the knee joint. The therapist then uses his or her own leg in a lunge position to support the weight of the client's leg. It may be helpful to ask the client to move toward the edge of the table or to lie on a diagonal.

To target the stretch for the gluteus medius muscle, flex the client's hip higher than the table and maintain the leg in a straight position while moving through adduction.

Be sure the client's pelvis is stabilized by stabilizing the knee of the uninvolved leg. If it isn't, the client's pelvis and lower torso will rotate toward the side where the leg is being stretched. This creates an illusion of greater range of motion and/or means the client will not experience a significant stretch in the abductor muscles.

The client may not feel a stretch in the intended muscle if his/her thighs are being compressed together, as that won't allow for full adduction. Try re-positioning the flexed leg so it is out of the way.

Hip Flexors—Rectus Femoris and Iliopsoas

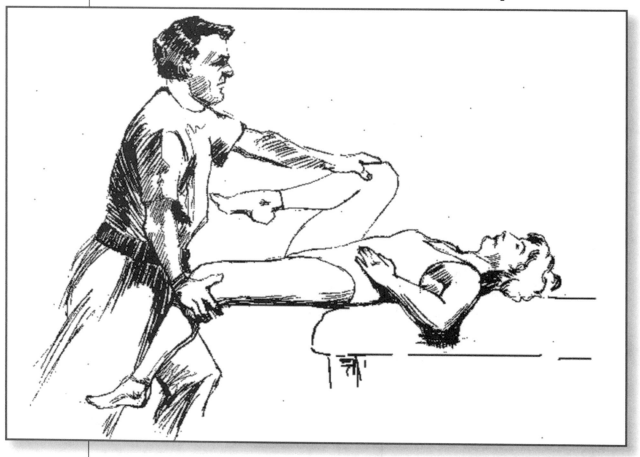

Client's Position

1. Begin with the client standing at the foot of the table.

2. The client places both ischial tuberosities on the very edge of the table.

3. The client flexes at the hip, placing both hands on the knee of the leg NOT being stretched.

4. The client leans back into a supine position, with the leg to be stretched hanging off the end of the table. The therapist can provide assistance to ensure the client's comfort and safety.

Passive Stretch Procedure

1. Stand in a lunge position facing the head of the table.

2. Stabilize the client's leg just proximal to the knee joint with your outside hand; be sure to bring the knee into a straight line with the client's hip.

3. Stabilize the client's other leg at the knee; be sure to keep the client's low back flat on the table by using your hand to 'push' that leg toward his/her head. This will posteriorly rotate the client's pelvis.

4. Extend the hip with your outside hand, pushing the leg toward the floor.

Considerations

You may ask the client to use both hands to hold his/her knee to the chest. If the client feels a pinching sensation in the hip of the opposite leg, ask him/her to stabilize the leg by grasping behind the upper thigh, just proximal to the knee.

Pectoralis Major

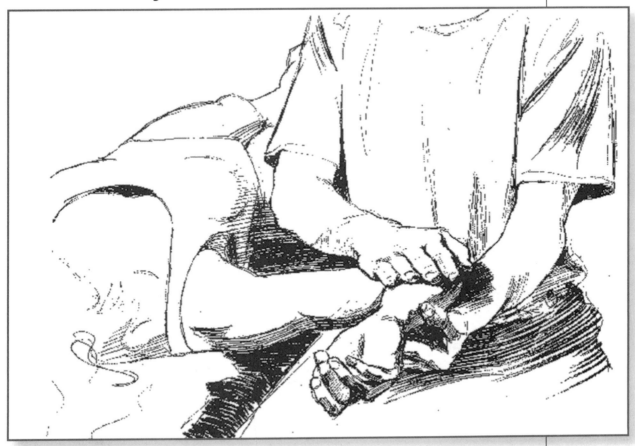

Client's Position

Supine and at the edge of the table. The arm is abducted and laterally rotated with the elbow flexed (as in a 'traffic cop' position). The shoulder joint must be even with, or just beyond the edge of, the table.

Passive Stretch Procedure

1. Kneel in a lunge position facing the head of the table.
2. Stabilize the forearm from beneath with your outside hand; your inside hand is placed proximal to the client's elbow from above—thus, your two hands face in opposition to each other.
3. Take the client's arm through extension and upward rotation of the scapula. You will be stretching the arm high over the client's head, while simultaneously pressing the client's arm toward the floor.

Considerations

Be sure the client does not feel any strain in the shoulder joint region. A stretch may be enhanced by asking the client to exhale the arm is being stretched. A stretch may be enhanced by placing a bolster or rolled-up towel under the client's shoulder.

Neck Flexion (Supporting Client's Shoulder)

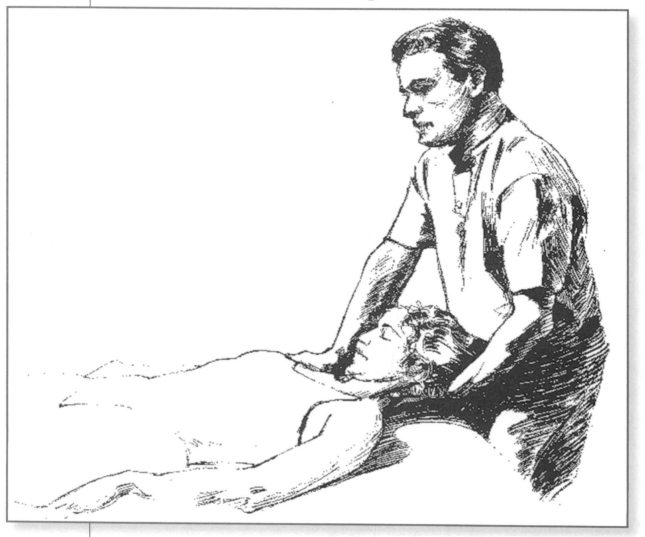

Client's Position

Supine and positioned at the end of the table to assist the therapist in maintaining proper body mechanics.

Passive Stretch Procedure

1. Stand at the head of the table in a lunge position.
2. Stabilize one shoulder against the table with your hand on the same side. Stabilize the neck and base of the head (occipital ridge) with your other hand.
3. Flex the neck in an arc-like fashion using your legs to create the movement. Avoid pinning the client's chin to his/her chest.

Considerations

This stretch can be performed with varying degrees of cervical rotation as well.

Neck Flexion (Arms Criss-Cross)

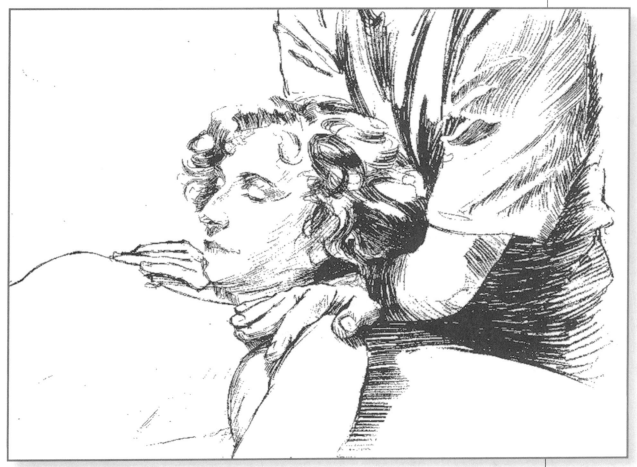

Client's Position

Supine and positioned at the end of the table to assist the therapist in maintaining proper body mechanics.

Passive Stretch Procedure

1. Stand at the head of the table in a lunge position or horse stance.

2. Stabilize the client's shoulders; use as much of your palms as possible. Position yourself low to the table so the client's head rests on your forearms. Your forearms are crossed behind the client's head.

3. Flex the client's neck in an arc-like fashion, using your legs to create the movement. Avoid pinning the client's head to his/her chest.

Neck Lateral Flexion (Arms Criss-Cross)

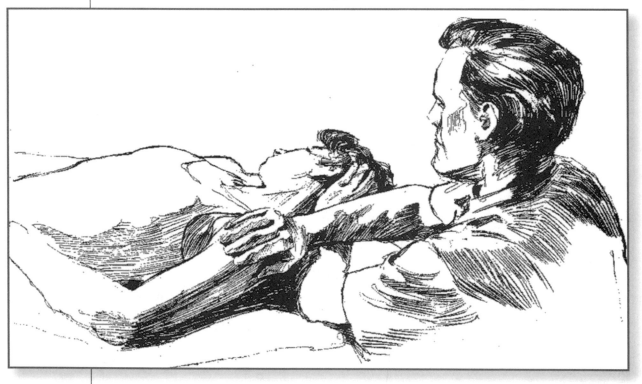

Client's Position

Supine with the neck rotated and laterally flexed away from the side being stretched.

Passive Stretch Procedure

1. Kneel at the side of the table.

2. By crossing your arms, stabilize the shoulder with your superior hand and stabilize the base of the head (occipital ridge) with your inferior hand.

3. Laterally flex the neck (with some rotation) in an arc-like fashion, away from the side where you are kneeling.

Considerations

You may enhance the stretch by either pushing the head further or depressing the shoulder more. Do not bend the head/neck all the way over to the opposite shoulder. The client may be hypo-mobile in the neck region, thus requiring additional shoulder depression.

Neck (Sidelying)

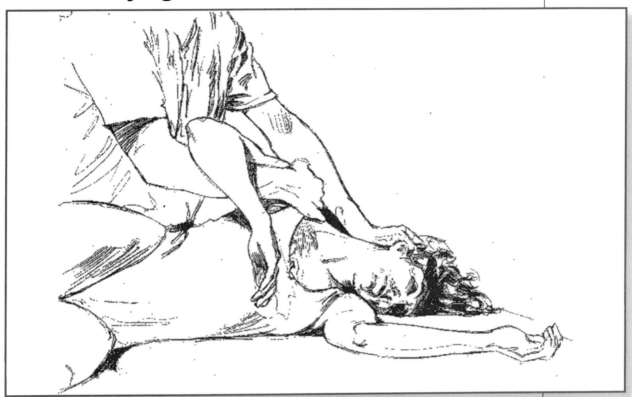

Client's Position

In a sidelying position, facing away from the therapist. The side to be stretched is on top. The client is at the edge of the table to assist the therapist in maintaining good body mechanics.

Passive Stretch Procedure

1. Stand in a lunge facing the head of the table.
2. Stabilize the top of the shoulder by cupping it with your inside/inferior hand, with the client's forearm/elbow overlapping your forearm/elbow. Your inside/inferior hand should be in front of the shoulder to be stretched.
3. Stabilize the lateral aspect of the occipital ridge with your outside/superior hand.
4. Depress the shoulder by pulling it down toward the client's feet. Use your hips to lean back and create the lift. Maintain the client's head in a stationary position.

Considerations

a. Be sure to keep the client's shoulders stacked. Rolling of the client's torso or shoulder may inhibit the desired stretch.
b. If the client experiences any pain, tingling or burning, stop and adjust the position of the head, or stop the stretch completely. This stretch can potentially cause unpleasant sensations in nerves or other tissues.
c. To isolate the posterior cervicals, stabilize the occipital ridge at mid-line with your outside/superior hand and add flexion of the neck while depressing the shoulder.
d. Do not over-flex the neck by pinning the client's chin to his/her chest.
e. Variations in the stretch may be obtained by rotating the head at different angles.

Latissimus Dorsi/Obliques (Sidelying)

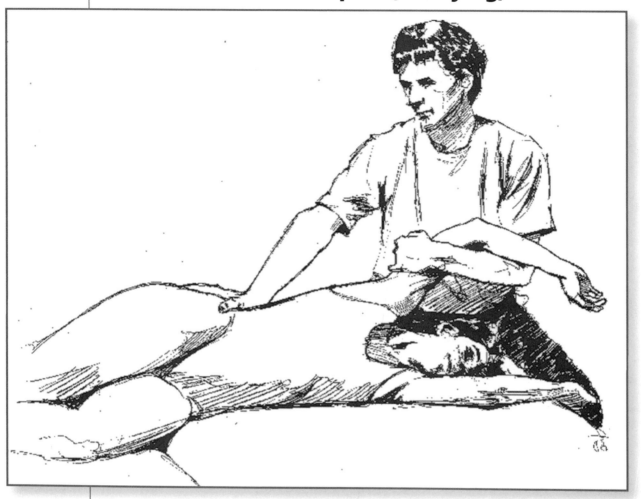

Client's Position

In a sidelying position, facing away from the therapist. The side to be stretched is on top. The client is at the edge of the table to assist the therapist in maintaining good body mechanics.

Passive Stretch Procedure

1. Stand in a lunge position facing the foot of the table.

2. Stabilize the top of the hip by cupping it with your outside/inferior hand.

3. Stabilize the arm with your inside/superior hand by overlapping your forearm/elbow with the client's forearm/elbow. Your inside/superior hand should be in front of the shoulder.

4. Depress the hip by pushing it down toward the client's feet, simultaneously pulling the client's arm overhead.

Considerations

a. Be sure the client's hips and shoulders stay stacked. Any rolling of the torso or shoulders may inhibit the stretch.

b. Ask the client to inhale when beginning the stretch. This will help expand the ribs.

OPTION: Allow the client's top leg to slightly hang off the table, while maintaining a straight torso. Therapist use a cross stretch position by standing behind the client, place the inferior hand on the client's scapula and place the superior hand on the client's hip, thus creating a criss cross of the therapist's arms. Apply a horizontal pressure to create stretch in the client's obliques.

Clinical Foundations

CLINICAL PROGRESSION VS. SWEDISH PROGRESSION

Clinical Progression uses all the same tools that the student has been practicing up to this time. A therapeutic progression looks very similar to a Swedish massage progression, but with a fundamental difference: the intent. The intent of a Swedish massage is to enhance circulation and promote relaxation. As you have already learned, a Swedish massage progression is:

ELEMENTS OF A SWEDISH MASSAGE PROGRESSION

1. Initial Contact
2. Warming
3. Assessment
4. Attending to a Specific Area
5. Circulatory/Draining
6. Transition or Completion

In contrast, the intent of a Clinical Progression is to assess soft tissue to locate areas of pathology and to facilitate change in that tissue to promote homeostasis. We use the word "facilitate" because we do not have the ability to 'cure' or 'heal' others. We, as massage therapists, are simply helping the body by encouraging its own self-healing.

ELEMENTS OF A CLINICAL PROGRESSION

1. Initial Contact
2. General Warming
3. Specific Warming
4. Specific Treatment
5. Muscular Lengthening
6. Transition or Completion

Know for midterm

ELEMENTS OF A CLINICAL PROGRESSION

1. Initial Contact

Initial contact in a clinical progression is much the same as in a Foundational progression, and refers to how one introduces touch to the receiver. This can apply to the first contact of the entire massage or can include initial contact to a new or different body area. In either case, the goal is to make initial contact in a way that is respectful and gives the receiver and his/her body an opportunity to become comfortable with your touch. A poor initial contact may result in the client becoming unreceptive to the work through armoring.

2. General Warming

In a clinical progression, general warming refers to the application of massage to a wide area for the purpose of assessment and preparation. The intent of general warming is to increase circulation and to begin to prepare the area by decreasing general muscle tension and increasing tissue receptivity. In a way, general warming is much like a pre-event sports massage without the intent to stimulate. Its goal is to bring the body into an optimal state for the specific activity to follow (namely, the application of specific therapeutic techniques).

Good general warming is essential for good assessment. Because of its diminished vascular circulation, ischemic tissue is much slower to warm than the surrounding tissues. As the surrounding tissues soften and become more pliable, differentiation between healthy and unhealthy soft tissue is enhanced. The harder, more resistant, ischemic tissues become more obvious. An example of general warming would be to apply any of the essential techniques to the entire back or entire low back.

3. Specific Warming

Specific warming contrasts from general warming in that it is focused on a specific muscle, muscle group, or smaller area. Its purpose is to assess and identify the exact location of pathology, i.e., ischemia, fibrosis, trigger points, tender points, etc., as well as prepare that site for the application of specific therapeutic techniques. An example of specific warming would be to apply short muscle strips to the longissimus lumborum or lumbar erector spinae.

4. Specific Treatment

The heart of the clinical progression is the application of specific therapeutic techniques with the focus of facilitating direct change in the physiology of unhealthy soft tissue. At this time we will focus on four primary tools:

a. Muscle stripping

b. Friction variations

c. Trigger point therapy

d. Myofascial therapy

Each of these techniques may and will be used at other points in the progression but will be used here for the direct purpose of creating change. Information regarding the benefit and specific application of each of these tools will be provided later in this lesson.

5. Muscular Lengthening

In order for pathological musculature to achieve its proper length, and therefore proper tonus, the muscle fibers must be lengthened. This can be achieved through the use of a wide variety of techniques. Two methods of lengthening generally used in a clinical progression are:

Gliding Techniques—The slow application of muscle stripping, forearm variations, and other gliding techniques used to bring length to soft tissues.

Stretching Techniques—Passive, as well as active-assisted, stretching (tense and relax, reciprocal inhibition, etc.). Stretching is essential for helping return muscle to its proper tonus. Stretching is especially important when treating trigger points.

6. Completion/Transition

As in a Swedish progression, completion and transition refers to how the massage therapist finishes work in one area and moves from that area to another. The goal is to let the client know that the treatment in one area is finished and to smoothly, with continuity, shift attention to a new area of focus to begin the therapeutic progression once again. Completion can also describe how the hands-on portion of a massage session is brought to a conclusion. Obviously, there are myriad ways in which both transition and completion can be accomplished.

Thermal Therapy Application

Enormous benefit can be derived from the application of heat or ice during or immediately following a clinical massage progression. Moist heat packs applied to an area previous to treatment can hasten the tissue warming process, save time and effort, and make the muscle, as well as other tissues, much more receptive to specific work.

Depending upon the type of specific treatment applied, heat or cold can be a necessary follow-up to the massage. When working with trigger points, chronically hypertonic musculature, or areas of ischemia, post-massage heat application will greatly increase the massage effectiveness and promote homeostasis. When dealing with fibrotic tissue, applying deep friction techniques, or any time the therapist may intentionally or unintentionally create trauma in the tissues, ice application immediately following treatment will help to counteract the body's inflammation response process and, thus, decrease recovery time and promote circulation.

Note: Although initial contact, general warming, specific warming, specific treatment, muscular lengthening, and transition/completion are the essential elements of a Clinical Progression, there are some other very important components that must be considered:

- Assessment
- Communication
- Thoroughness
- The variable order of the progression

COMPONENTS OF A CLINICAL PROGRESSION

In addition to the six elements, there are some very important components of a Clinical Progression.

Assessment

Assessment is the educated evaluation of tissue and treatment effectiveness. In a Clinical Progression, assessment is a constant. The state and health of the soft tissues are being attended to throughout every part of a Clinical Progression. This can apply to any pre- 'hands on' questioning, analysis, or muscle testing, as well as during the massage treatment. Assessment skills are used to locate areas of pathology by discerning differences between healthy and unhealthy tissues, or between those that are very unhealthy and those that are somewhat less unhealthy. Assessment is also used following specific treatment to gauge the degree of change in the tissues, and to determine if the treatment has been successful.

The Order of Elements in a Clinical Progression

Within a Clinical Progression there is constant movement between the different parts of the progression. A therapist can move from any part of the progression to a previous segment at any time. For example, one can move from specific treatment to general warming, or from lengthening to specific warming, etc.

Thoroughness

When treating specific conditions or pathologies or using a Clinical Progression, it becomes very important to be thorough in both assessment and treatment. Not only should the specific site of a problem be addressed, but so should nearby related areas, muscles which are antagonistic to those that are problematic, and all parts of the affected muscle: the belly, bony attachments, and tendons. Only in this way can a therapist be sure to help create conditions for the body to return to homeostasis. Otherwise, the condition or pathology may return.

In order to do a complete Clinical Progression, the student needs to:

- Ask the client to perform an appropriate action to contract the muscle.
- Palpate and apply specific therapeutic techniques to the muscle and musculotendinous unit.
- Palpate and apply specific therapeutic techniques to the muscle attachment sites.

Communication

The intent and specificity of a Clinical Progression necessitates greater involvement of the client and, as a result, places greater importance on communication between the client and the therapist. Unlike a Swedish progression where the therapist wants to disrupt the client as little as possible, in a Clinical Progression both the therapist and the client must maintain constant attention to the process of finding and treating pathological tissue, primarily through communication. This heightened communication can be categorized into three types: verbal, visual, and tactile.

Verbal Communication—Prior to the treatment, questioning about client history, activities, and the etiology of specific conditions will help focus the massage treatment, saving time and energy and increasing effectiveness. During the treatment, frequent questioning of the client about his/her experience (i.e., discomfort levels, types of pain, referral sensations, and the specific location of problems) is essential for good assessment and treatment.

Visual and tactile communication are important as well. Observing client responses via visual cues (grimaces, twitches, breath, etc.) and tactile cues (jump signs, armoring, spasms, etc.) can often provide as much information as verbal responses. The therapist should remain ever vigilant in attentiveness to these cues.

THE FEEL OF THE TISSUES

Tissues May Be Classified in 2 Ways

- Hard tissues (cartilage, bone)
- Soft tissues (skin, fascia, muscles, tendons, ligaments)

Tissues May Be Normal or Abnormal

- Each tissue has a particular feel under normal conditions.
- Each tissue may have varying degrees of altered feel depending upon the pathology.

Normal

- This is an individual matter. All normal tissues do not have the same feel. For example: athlete vs. society matron; Other examples: age, amount of physical activity, genetics, nutrition or sleep.
- These all present varying degrees of resistance, resiliency or tone each of which would be 'normal' for the individual.
- To determine the normal under all conditions takes time and the education of your hands.
- Variations from normal may be in the direction of tensed or relaxed tissues.
- The more tense the tissues, the easier it will be to distinguish from normal.

Living Things (Tissues > Cells) Prefer

- Persuasion vs. force
- Consideration vs. trauma
- Intelligence vs. ill expended energy
- Less vs. more

It Is Better To Work WITH the Tissues Rather Than AT the Tissues

Technique follows perception.
What you imagine is what you touch.

STRATEGIES FOR PERFORMING CLINICAL MASSAGE THERAPY

How to Develop Palpation Skills

- Be present and aware.

- Slow down and quiet your body and mind to 'listen.' Use all of your sensing tools.

- Calm your breath; relax your shoulders, arms and hands. A therapist will feel less the more tension is held in his/her body.

- Disguise all palpation as massage. Make it a part of your session, not separate from it.

- Sink slowly into tissues to engage. Remember, most muscles are superficial. You do not need to 'dig in.' Avoid excessive pressure. Less is more.

- Don't look intently on the area; rather, look away.

- Use an easy, moderate-tempo, broad friction sweep with finger pads. Do not jab or poke the tissue.

- Create a dialogue of what you are feeling in the tissue . . . verbally, visually and kinesthetically.

- Intentionally apply the quality of your touch through the technique.

- Technique is a language we use to communicate with the body. It is not necessarily the technique that will create the change, but rather, the quality of how you applied the technique . . . how you touch.

> To force someone's process is the worst thing you can do.

Communication

- Effective communication is an important part of effective clinical work.

- You do not have to have all the answers.

- Allow your clients to help you direct the session by the way they answer your questions.

- Ask specific/closed-ended questions vs. general/open-ended questions to help direct your session.

General/Open Ended Questions vs. Specific/Closed-Ended Questions

General/Open Ended Questions	Specific/Closed-Ended Questions
Is the pressure ok?	Is this too much or too little pressure?
How's the pressure?	Does this feel effective?
How does this feel?	Is this area tender, sensitive, sore?
Does this feel OK?	Which feels like it's creating more relief: 1, 2 or 3?
Do you have any contraindications?	Would you like more time spent here or to move on?

Specific OPPQRST Questions For the Client

O	Onset	When does it happen?
P	Provoking	What sets it off?
P	Palliative	What makes it feel better?
Q	Quality of Pain	Nervy, throbbing, dull, muscular, sharp?
R	Radiates	Does it? If so, where?
S	Site of Pain	Where?
T	Timing	AM or PM?

CONDITIONS IN SOFT TISSUE AFFECTING TISSUE HEALTH

Adhesion

The binding of adjacent layers of soft tissue, i.e., two or more muscles, layers in muscle, or muscle fibers; fascia and muscle; or fascial layers. Typically indicates tissue ischemia, dehydration, or thickening. Tends to inhibit free movement of muscle and fascia and hence leads to pain, muscle imbalance, dysfunction, and postural distortion.

Fibrosis (Fibrotic Buildup)

The formation of fibrous tissue as a reparative or reactive process, as opposed to the formation of fibrous tissue as a normal constituent of an organ or tissue (Steadman's). Refers to the formation of scar tissue and/or fibrotic buildup (fibroblast cells in connective tissue laying down additional matrix) in an area it does not normally occur as part of a healing, supportive, or protective process.

Lesion

A circumscribed area of pathologically altered tissue (Taber's). Lesions in soft tissue can result from strain (tearing), inordinate stress, tissue trauma, or other disease processes, and can include tissue changes from the inflammatory or healing processes. Lesions are characterized in two types:

1. **Primary Lesion:** the direct result of injury or disease, i.e., a tear in the tissue.

2. **Secondary Lesion:** the result of the primary lesion and the body's response to it, i.e., scar tissue.

Ischemia

Ischemia is the lack of blood flow through an area or tissue. Can potentially be due to many factors such as hypertonicity, vascular constriction, fibrosis, adhesion, vascular entrapment, vascular disease, injury or secondary injury. Potentially results in pain, cell necrosis, and resistance to healing.

Trigger Points

See the Trigger Point section in this manual.

Strain

Trauma to a muscle or musculotendinous unit due to excessively violent contraction or excessively forceful stretch.

The term "strain" can also be applied to injuries not associated with sudden trauma:

1. **Repetitive Strain:** Also referred to as a repetitive motion injury, a repetitive strain is an injury to soft tissue resulting from the repeated performance of an activity or action.

2. **Concentric Strain (adaptive shortening):** Concentric strain is an injury to muscle tissue resulting from prolonged hypertonicity and sustained contraction and shortening of the fibers.

3. **Eccentric Strain (adaptive lengthening):** Eccentric strain is an injury in muscle tissue resulting from prolonged hypotonicity and sustained contraction in an elongated state.

CAUSAL FACTORS

Definition: "That which has an effect on tissue, movement, or body alignment."

Two Types of Causal Factors

1. Perpetuating Factors

- Conditions or situations that can be altered or changed.

- These conditions or situations contribute to the enhancement of any signs and symptoms of pain or discomfort.

- Conditions resulting in pain or discomfort may take a long time to correct, depending on how long the condition and the causal factors contributing to the condition have existed.

2. Predisposing Factors

- Conditions or situations that cannot be permanently changed.

- These conditions or situations precede the signs and symptoms of pain.

- Predisposing factors do not mean a person must continually experience pain; however, an ongoing maintenance program might need to be implemented in order for the person to be pain-free.

- Taber's Dictionary: "indicating a tendency to, susceptibility to."

Additional Terms

These terms are also used to describe types of perpetuating and predisposing factors:

- **Structural (causes or factors):** That which is affected by bone, ligament. These are difficult to change.

- **Functional (causes or factors):** Affected by soft tissues—muscles, tendons, aponeurosis, superficial and deep fascia. Adaptable, conforms, and is highly changeable.

- **Biomechanical stress area:**

  - Bony structure where two or more muscles attach, resulting in two or more directions of tensile pull.

  - Muscles that cross more than one joint

Muscle Stripping

MUSCLE STRIPPING

Muscle stripping is a deep, specific gliding stroke applied with the direction of the muscle fibers. Often the stroke will proceed along the length of the muscle from one attachment to the other, but shorter strokes can also be used. Depending on the speed and depth at which it is applied, it can have differing effects.

It is especially effective in creating change in chronic injury patterns, often alleviating a condition your client has lived with for many years. For active clients, muscle stripping helps keep tissue healthy and the client at peak performance.

Therefore, muscle stripping can be used for a variety of purposes, depending upon how it is applied. An important variable in muscle stripping application is the speed or pacing of the stroke.

- **Fast muscle stripping**—tends to be lighter in pressure and engagement, and is most effective as a specific warming stroke. As the muscle warms and softens, engagement depth increases, and the stroke gradually begins to decrease in speed.

- **Slow muscle stripping**—most often used as a lengthening stroke to effectively reduce tension. Deeper engagement into the muscle in combination with a more engaged 'stretch' of the muscle as the technique glides, can help reduce a muscle's tendency towards contraction or hypertonicity.

- **Moderate speed muscle stripping**—somewhere between fast and slow muscle stripping. A muscle stripping stroke of moderate speed is very useful as an assessment stroke. As the practitioner glides 'through' the muscle tissue at a moderate speed, differentiation between areas of health and pathology will become apparent. Pathological areas will often be described as "stuck" or as "speed bumps." Ischemia in the muscles will make specific areas less pliable or 'giving' as the stroke passes through. A stroke of a faster speed would simply fly over these areas. A slow stroke would allow too much time for the unhealthy areas to move out of the way.

A good general rule is "the deeper the stroke, the slower the stroke." Although some clients can tolerate this deep work at a rapid speed, you usually want to move slowly enough to allow the muscle time to stretch, and to allow yourself time to feel whether you need to make micro-adjustments in your depth. Since you are working deeply, you will want to pull back occasionally and smooth out the area, allowing the client to relax and absorb the changes, before moving in again.

Try experimenting with different speed strokes and find what works best for different purposes.

Muscle Stripping as a Specific Therapeutic Tool

Muscle stripping can be a very valuable tool to help facilitate change in unhealthy muscle tissue. Specific short muscle stripping strokes are very effective at both lengthening and creating local hyperemia in the muscle. Here's how it works:

> As the therapist compresses into the muscle and begins the stroke, blood and other tissue fluid is being pushed out of the muscle. As the stroke begins to move in the direction of the muscle fibers, the continual compression pushes fluid out of new areas of the tissue, creating a wave of tissue and fluid directly ahead of it. Directly behind the area of compression, tissue and fluid are rushing back in to fill the void left as the compressive force moves. Also, the tissue fibers are being pulled taut and are thereby being lengthened, normalizing muscle tonus. This combination of circulatory effect and lengthening gives muscle stripping its great effectiveness.

Proper Application of Muscle Stripping

In order for a muscle stripping stroke to be effective, it has to be properly applied. To be effective, you must be able to sink into the tissue to the desired depth and compress the muscle before beginning your stroke.

1. **Muscle Stripping Tools**—Effective muscle stripping requires a small area of contact. Thumbs and fingers are the most commonly used tools because they not only allow for a specific stroke, but also afford the most sensitivity in reading the tissue response.

2. **Body and Hand Mechanics**—Good muscle stripping can be applied with either of two tools: thumb or fingertip. Whichever tool you use, make certain that the technique is applied with good body and hand mechanics.

   ■ Fingers or thumbs should be in direct alignment with the forearm.

   ■ The wrist should be in a neutral position—neither flexed nor extended.

   ■ Use a forward movement of your hips to help 'push' the strip along.

   ■ Any arm movement should be directed away from the center of your body.

3. **Bracing**—It is usually (but not necessarily always) best to assist your stripping tool by bracing it with some other tool. This can increase your pressure and control, and help prevent injury to your hands. Braced thumbs working together, fingertips of one hand directly on top of the fingertips of the other hand, and fingertips bracing a thumb are some examples. Experiment with different variations to find out what works best for you.

4. **Muscle Stripping Stroke Profile**— A properly applied muscle stripping stroke can be broken into two parts: the compression or engagement phase, and the gliding phase. The overall profile of the stroke looks something like an "L."

   Lift off the engagement at the end of the stroke.

   Caution: Be sure to compress into the muscle before beginning the glide. This is necessary to ensure good engagement. A common mistake is to begin gliding before engaging into the tissue, resulting in a stroke profile shaped like a "U." A U-shaped profile will often feel 'gouging' and is not effective.

   1. Engagement
   Compress into the muscle with the desired pressure and depth.

   2. Gliding
   Push through the muscle tissue in the direction of the muscle fibers maintaining the same level of depth.

   Important note: Be sure to differentiate your muscle stripping from a thumb-over-thumb or fingertip-over-fingertip effleurage. They are very different techniques and can have very different purposes and degrees of effectiveness.

   As with all gliding strokes, when working on the extremities, always perform this stroke towards the heart.

5. **Length of Stroke**—When beginning to learn this stroke, you will have the easiest time maintaining an effective depth and good mechanics if you limit the stroke to about 5–6 inches. As you gain proficiency you can vary the length of the stroke depending on your therapeutic intent, the length of the muscle, and tissue response.

6. **Therapeutic Effectiveness**—In order to get the desired change in the tissue, it is necessary to repeat a stroke a number of times. This includes several strokes for **assessment** purposes and to get the client comfortable with the stroke. Further repetitions will allow you to then work for the desired change.

Friction

FRICTION

The Use of Friction Techniques

During a Clinical Progression, friction techniques are invaluable. Different variations of friction are used primarily for three different purposes: muscle identification, assessment, and the treatment of soft tissue pathology, adhesions, fibrosis, pain, tenderness, or decreased range of movement.

- **Muscle Identification**—As a result of their increasing anatomical knowledge, students will be able to identify specific muscles by palpating the direction of their muscle fibers. By learning the origin, insertion, and fiber direction of a specific muscle, friction strokes can be utilized to identify the muscle, no matter its depth. A muscle's location and fiber direction will clearly differentiate it from other muscles. Circular fingertip friction is a good tool to locate a muscle. Cross-fiber (transverse) friction is great for ultimately determining fiber direction.

- **Assessment**—Friction strokes can also be used to help determine the location and state of unhealthy soft tissue. Areas of discomfort and, therefore, pathology can be readily identified using friction. Friction, especially cross-fiber friction, will help the therapist to locate the exact site of a problem.

- **Fibrotic Tissues and Adhesions**—Fibrotic buildup and adhesion are the common result of injury, chronic hypertonicity, and ischemia. Friction variations are great tools for breaking up scar tissue, 'unsticking' muscle and fascial layers, and creating the minute trauma necessary to bring blood (traumatic hyperemia) to the area for proper healing. Once broken up, scar tissue fibers can be encouraged to seek proper alignment with longitudinal (or with-the-fiber) friction. It is important to realign scar tissue so that it no longer interferes with normal function.

Friction is any technique in which the superficial tissues are pinned in place by the therapist's hand or fingers and thus moved over the underlying tissues/structures. Therefore, the most important characteristics of friction strokes are that they do not glide on the skin, that they affect the deeper layers of tissue, and that they are applied specifically to the affected area.

1. **Identification**
   - Fiber direction
   - Layering
   - Location
   - Quality of surrounding tissue

2. **Loosening**
   - Circulatory
   - Tissue preparation
   - Tissue receptivity
   - Chronic constriction
   - Transitional stroke
   - Feels good

3. **Breakdown**
   - Adhesion
   - Scar tissue
   - Fibrotic tissue
   - Prevent formation and laying down of scar tissue

Variations of Friction Strokes

There are basically three varieties of specific friction strokes: circular, cross-fiber, and longitudinal.

- **Circular Friction**—Although it can be performed with the thumb, circular friction is most commonly applied with fingertips. It is a great stroke for initially differentiating muscle bellies and layers and for releasing adhesions, creating movement between those layers.

- **Cross-Fiber Friction**—Cross-fiber friction (XFF) is characterized by its angle of application. Cross-fiber friction is always applied at a 90-degree angle, or perpendicular to the muscle fiber direction. As mentioned above, cross-fiber friction is the best friction tool for assessment and for breaking up fibrosis and adhesion.

  NOTE: Cross-fiber friction can be the most invasive and irritating of the friction strokes and should be used with deference. If your client experiences too much discomfort with cross-fiber friction, switch to one of the other friction variations or use another technique.

■ **Longitudinal Friction**—Longitudinal friction is characterized by its angle of application as well. The stroke is applied in the same direction as (parallel to) the muscle fibers. This variation is good for breaking up adhesions as well, and is a good alternative if cross-fiber friction is too invasive. Longitudinal friction, as mentioned above, is good for helping encourage the realignment of scar tissue.

As already described, friction can be a very intense and irritating stroke to receive. It is best to periodically interrupt friction techniques with other techniques which are "feel good" in nature.

One-Directional vs. Two-Directional Friction Strokes

Transverse and longitudinal friction techniques can be performed with the engagement of the stroke applied in either one direction or back and forth in two directions. When using a cross-fiber friction, it may be best to apply the force of the friction in one direction only. Why? A properly applied friction stroke in a single direction separates and spreads fibers in one direction, lightens up the pressure without breaking contact with the skin, and returns to the starting position to get set to engage and friction again. This brief break between strokes allows blood to come into the area and offers a respite from any discomfort the client may be experiencing. A two-directional cross-fiber friction, as a result of the repetition, tends to feel like 'sawing' back and forth and can be very irritating to the client, as well as injurious to the therapist. When applying longitudinal friction, a two-directional friction stroke is not as invasive or uncomfortable, and can be useful in realigning muscle fibers.

Principles of Applying Effective Cross-Fiber Friction

1. Done only after thoroughly warming tissues.
2. Applied at the exact site and correct angle to those fibers.
3. Emphasize engagement and feeling of the tissue.
4. Slow down and gradually melt down into tissues to reach the appropriate depth.
5. Applied with the therapist's tool, skin and underlying tissues moving as one unit.
6. Use pads, not tips, of thumb or fingers.
7. Avoid joints hyperextending.
8. Use your center to engage the tissue to keep the hands and arms relaxed.
9. Use of a broad transverse sweep appropriate to the width of the muscle working. Keep the pressure consistent throughout the stroke. Most XFF strokes are performed in one direction.
10. Do not GLIDE across tissue. Do not use too much oil, as it will prevent the therapist from engaging the tissues.
11. Avoid flipping abruptly over fiber bands.
12. Done with muscle or tissue in a relaxed position, except with a sheathed tendon, which is done in a stretched (taut) position.
13. Applied frequently enough to have a progressive impact on the adhered tissue.
14. Followed by ice application for 10–15 minutes.
15. Apply movement with the involved musculature after ice application.

APPLICATION OF CROSS-FIBER FRICTION FOLLOWING INJURY

Definitions of Stages of Inflammation

- Acute: in an injury, usually the first 24 hours. The site is red, hot, swollen and painful.

- Subacute: usually 48–76 hours after an injury where the swelling, though still present and painful, is not increasing.

- Chronic: usually at least 76 hours after the original injury; this stage can last continuously or intermittently for weeks, months or years. The site may not be visibly swollen, but will often be somewhat painful and maintain some loss of function.

Level I–II Strain

1. Acute (24–48 hours)
   a. No cross-fiber
   b. RICE (Rest, Ice, Compression, Elevation) application
   c. No movement
   d. Proximal to area: light stroking
   e. General relaxation to the rest of the body

2. Subacute (48–76 hours)
   a. No cross-fiber
   b. RICE application
   c. Movement, via gentle pain-free cryokinetics
   d. Proximal to area: effleurage/pétrissage
   e. Injury site: light compression and stroking
   f. General relaxation to rest of body

3. Chronic (after 76 hours)
   a. Cross-fiber 2–6 minutes (less depth required for level 1)
   b. Ice application follows
   c. Pain free isometric contraction and active ROM
   d. Frequency: 1–2 times per week for 1–2 weeks. 1 time per week for up to 4 weeks.

Level III Strain

1. Acute (24–76 hours)
   a. Follow guidelines as above for use of RICE only for 24–76 hours.
   b. Essential to have suspected Level III strain evaluated by medical personnel and to coordinate massage treatment jointly.

2. Chronic (72+ hours)
   a. Initiation of any massage treatment will depend upon: extent of inflammation, discoloration, presence of contusion or hematoma, and evaluation by medical personnel.
   b. Cross-fiber friction 5–10 minutes per site.
   c. Ice application. Ice may also be used prior to cross-fiber friction for an analgesic effect.
   d. No movement to be utilized with a recent Level III strain where there is any possibility of trauma and/or reinjury to the site. Therefore, use of movement may be restricted to cryokinetics longer, and will often be initiated later, than with a Level I or II strain.
   e. Frequency: May require 2–3 applications per week for 2 weeks; 1–2 applications per week for 2–3 additional weeks.

Long-Term Scar Tissue

(Present at least 8 weeks; tissue highly contracted; more palpable scarring)

1. Length of treatment per site will range from 6–15 minutes depending upon the extent and longevity of scarring.

2. Work transversely in one direction only, to provide more comfort for client and therapist.

3. Active ROM and resisted movement to follow ice application.

4. Frequency: 2 times per week for 3–6 weeks. Treatments taper off as ROM increases and inflammation decreases.

5. Deep tissue/fascial lengthening critical in longer-term injuries to scarred and surrounding areas.

6. Employment of corrective exercise is also vital.

Goals/Physiological Effects

- To break up scar tissue/adhesions by mimicking the shortening, broadening action of the contracting muscle.
- To facilitate full ROM by restoring the normal parallel direction of the muscle's fibers.
- To increase circulation (venous and lymphatic) in ischemic tissues affected by scarring.
- To prevent extraneous scar tissue formation in recent soft tissue injuries.
- To free capillary flow in the layers of connective tissue.
- To continually clear areas of biomechanical stress and strain common to the athlete in maintenance massage.
- To warm and loosen the muscle and connective tissues in general.

Indications

- Muscle strain (subacute/chronic)
- Sprain (subacute/chronic)
- Scar tissue/adhesions
- Tendonitis
- Fasciitis
- Chronic contracture of soft tissue
- General massage, loosening and warm-up
- Lesion at musculoskeletal juncture
- Tenosynovitis
- Recent trauma

Contraindications

- Muscle strain/sprain (acute & subacute, see notes)
- Pre-event/Post-event (deep work)
- Inflammation due to bacterial or viral infection
- Osteoarthritis (active phase)
- Rheumatoid arthritis any time
- Bursitis
- Lesion over nerve plexus
- Ossification of ligament

Proprioceptive Techniques

Trigger Point Treatment Recap

- Warm Tissue
- Could use multidemensional skin rolling or myofacial techniques
  - Trigger point therapy
  - Stretch tissue
  - Moist Heat 10 - 20 minutes

NEUROMUSCULAR RELEASE (NMR)

Indications for Neuromuscular Release

- Any technique that is directed at decreasing muscle tension and/or spasms that restrict ROM and/or make movement painful.

- Many physiological processes are involved in the development of general tension, pain and hypersensitive points within muscles; therefore, combining interventions can be used to address the problem.

- NMR can be used anytime an athlete has limited and/or painful movement, as a way to effectively normalize muscle tone.

Contraindications for Neuromuscular Release

- Acute stage musculoskeletal injury because of splinting

- Acute swelling/inflammation

- Open wounds

- Local infection

- Acute rheumatoid arthritis

- Malignancy

3 Categories of Neuromuscular Release

1. Proprioceptive techniques
2. Positional release
3. Trigger point

PROPRIOCEPTIVE TECHNIQUES

There are a variety of proprioceptive techniques, which combine muscle contraction and movement to create enhanced joint mobility, decrease muscle tension and splinting, and increase resting length. Using these techniques in conjunction with your other techniques can increase the effectiveness of all your work. Proprioceptive techniques utilize the proprioceptive reflexes to bring about the desired change, hence the name. Proprioceptive techniques are characterized by the following:

- Use active muscle contraction to decrease muscle tension by stimulating specific neuromuscular reflexes that control muscle tone

- Designed to decrease movement barriers related to muscle and fascial tension

- Goals are to inhibit muscle spasms that restrict ROM and cause pain, and to enhance the effectiveness of trigger point and positional release techniques

While there are many variations, we will be focusing on two: **contract-relax** and **reciprocal inhibition.** Both of these techniques come from Proprioceptive Neuromuscular Facilitation (PNF), but have elements in common with most of the proprioceptive techniques.

When incorporated into your clinical progression, the proprioceptive techniques can greatly enhance the overall effectiveness of your work. These techniques have great benefit if you are working with athletes; they can reduce muscle spasm and shortens post-event and are great tools to use during the maintenance phase as athletes engage in various stretching programs. These benefits are true for the less athletic as well. As they work with the nervous system they are also great tools to help with neuromuscular re-education, which retrains the muscles and nervous systems in regards to muscle tension and length. A final benefit to the therapist is it can be done while the client is clothed, which can come in handy in many situations.

CONTRACT RELAX

Contract-Relax Theory

The exact physiology of how contract-relax works is a hotly debated subject. But while the exact mechanism is not agreed upon, what seems to be clear is that it uses the principle of post-isometric relaxation (PIR). (Please note that there is a proprioceptive technique that uses the same name.) This principle states that: "Following on from an isometric contraction . . . there is a refractory, or latency, period of approximately 15 seconds during which there can be an easier (due to reduced tone) movement towards the new position (new resistance barrier) of a joint or muscle" (JBMT 01/2002 or Chaitow 1996 *Muscle Energy Techniques*). Or, as Cash states:

> Immediately following a period of isometric contraction, a muscle becomes inhibited and more relaxed (hypotonic) for about 5–10 seconds before its normal tone returns. During this induced period of deep relaxation the tissues can be passively stretched further and held in this new position for 10–15 seconds, to allow the nervous system to accept the new tissue length. The increased elasticity achieved by this will be permanent, providing the original cause of the problem (shortening) has been resolved and stretching exercises are performed for a few days. (Cash 1996: 206)

The result is that the client receives more effective stretching and the nervous system is allowed to reset. In this case, resetting means that the proprioceptors, particularly the muscle spindles, identify the increased length as normal.

Indications

- Muscle shortness and/or tension
- Postural imbalances
- Neuromuscular re-education
- Muscle spasm

Contraindications

- There are very few contraindications for this technique. As long as the client can safely move a joint and the contract-relax movements do not cause pain, then it can be used.

PROCEDURE FOR CONTRACT-RELAX TECHNIQUE

There are variations in descriptions of how to perform the contract-relax technique. These are mainly in how long to hold the contraction, how many times to repeat the contraction, the breathing pattern, and how long to hold the final stretch. The following procedure is described here as a starting point for learning the technique.

General Contract-Relax Protocol

1. Place the client in the correct position for the desired stretch. This is determined by the target muscle, the best ways to stretch it, and any client needs.

2. Determine the client's ROM for the targeted muscle or muscle group through a passive stretch. Feel for the motion barrier, or end-point, of the stretch. This step may also be accomplished by instructing the client to stretch actively.

3. Slowly move the target muscle into a stretched position, feeling for a motion barrier or slight tissue resistance. This should be pain-free, and the client may begin to feel a stretch. Do not move too quickly or too far, so as not to stimulate the stretch reflex.

4. At the motion barrier, instruct the receiver to contract against the resistance you provide. Ask the receiver to utilize a maximum of 20–30% of his or her muscle power. You meet the contraction with equal resistance. This will result in an **isometric** contraction. Hold for approximately 8 seconds as the client breathes normally.

5. Then, cue the client to relax fully. Ask the client to take a deep, relaxing breath. The therapist should feel the muscle let go and relax fully.

6. On the client's exhalation, the therapist moves the client to the next motion barrier or next place of slight tissue resistance.

7. Repeat steps 4–6 three to five times. End by taking the client to the next motion barrier and hold the last position for 20–30 seconds. Once in the final stretch position have the client breathe and focus his/her awareness on the target muscle.

If a client feels pain during this technique, there are several ways to modify it to keep it pain-free. Making sure the technique is performed pain free is very important, because pain tends to elicit a contraction/protective response which is counter to our goals.

- If a client feels pain when moving to a motion barrier, you can modify by moving less far and finding a more subtle motion barrier.

- If the client feels pain during the contraction phase, have him/her use less effort.

- If neither of these things work for decreasing the pain, try reciprocal inhibition (discussed next).

- If you cannot find a way to do it pain-free, then stop and try a different technique.

TIPS AND COMMON ERRORS FOR CONTRACT-RELAX

Tips for Applying the Techniques

- Place the body in the correct anatomical position for safety and to elicit the most effective isometric contraction.
- Make sure the client is relaxed and the joints are well supported throughout the procedure.
- Avoid pain by gently approaching the motion barrier or end point of the stretch.
- Instruct the client to breathe throughout the technique.
- Emphasize that only 20–30% of the client's muscle power should be used against the resistance, and that the contraction should be steady—not a 'muscle contest' like arm-wrestling.
- The isometric contraction should be introduced slowly, and resisted without any jerking, wobbling, or bouncing. (Chaitow 1997: 50)
- Give clear verbal instructions and maintain eye contact with the receiver.

Common Errors Made by *Clients* Performing Contract-Relax Techniques

(Chaitow 1997: 52)

- Contraction is too hard (more than 20–30% effort).
- Contraction is in the wrong direction.
- Contraction is not sustained long enough.
- Receiver does not relax completely after the contraction.
- Starting and/or finishing the contraction too hastily.

Clear instructions, repeating instructions, and patiently talking the receiver through the technique usually solves these problems.

Common Errors Made by *Practitioners* Applying Contract-Relax Techniques

(Chaitow 1997: 52)

- Inaccurate control of position of joint or muscle in relation to the resistance barrier.
  Remedy: have a clear image of what is required and apply it accordingly.
- Inadequate counterforce to the contraction.
  Remedy: meet and match the force to produce an isometric contraction (i.e., no movement).
- Counterforce is applied in an inappropriate direction.
  Remedy: identify the precise direction needed for the best effect.
- Moving to a new position too hastily after the contraction (there are about 25 seconds in which to apply the stretch after a contraction; haste is unnecessary and may be counter-productive).
- Inadequate or unclear instructions given to the receiver.
  Remedy: practice being precise, concise, and accurate.

Contract-Relax For Specific Muscles

For all contract-relax stretches there is the contraction phase and the stretch phase. For each of the following muscles they are identified separately for clarity. Remember to communicate clearly with your clients as you perform each procedure. For most muscles there may be many ways to perform the contract-relax stretching. Common and effective ways for each muscle are on the following pages.

Gastrocnemius/Soleus (Pushing)

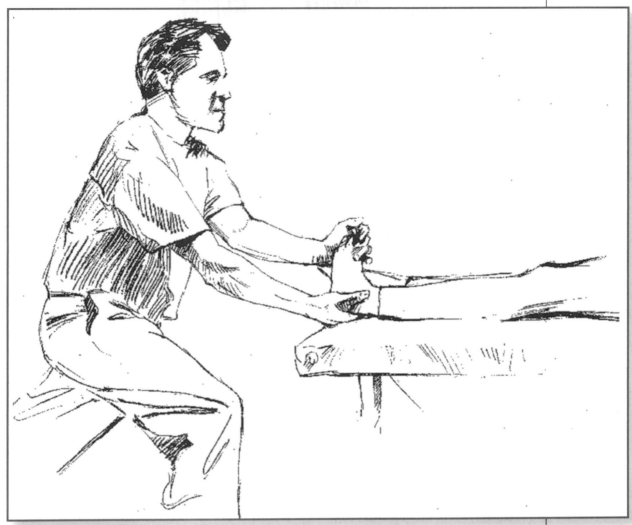

Contract-Relax Procedure

Contraction Phase

Ask your client to press (plantarflex) the ankle/foot away from the table. Standing in a lunge position, provide resistance with your hand.

Stretch Phase

1. Stabilize the ankle with your outside hand supporting the lateral malleolus and your inside hand at the ball of the foot.
2. Dorsiflex at the ankle toward the client's head.

Gastrocnemius/Soleus (Pulling)

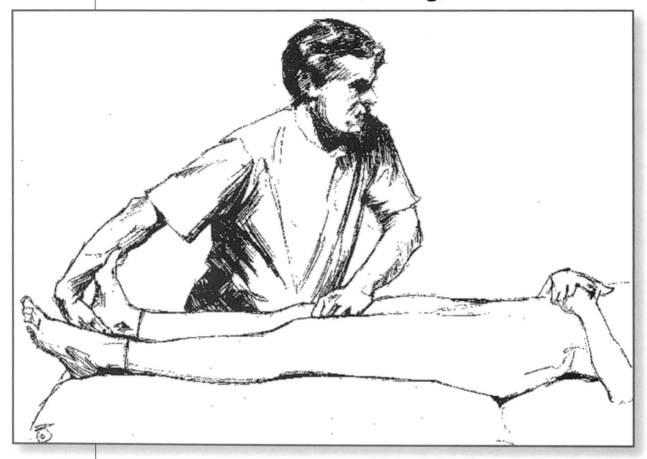

Contract-Relax Procedure

Contraction Phase

Ask your client to press (plantarflex) the ankle/foot away from the table. Standing in a lunge position, provide resistance with your forearm.

Stretch Phase

1. Stabilize the foot/ankle with your inside/inferior hand with the client's heel in your palm and the client's ball of the foot against your forearm. Stabilize the leg proximal to the knee joint with your outside/superior hand.

   Caution: Avoid hyperextension of the knee joint.

2. Dorsiflex the ankle toward the client's head using your weight and leverage from the lunge position.

Hamstrings (Straight Leg)

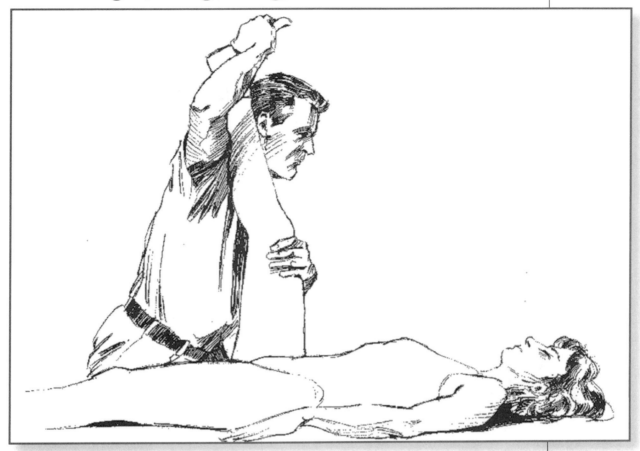

Contract-Relax Procedure

Contraction Phase

Ask your client to press (extend) the straight leg toward the table. From a lunge position, provide resistance with your shoulder.

Stretch Phase

1. Stabilize the client's straight leg just proximal to the knee joint with your outside hand; the inside hand is placed behind the client's ankle or over the ball of the foot.

2. Flex the hip in an arc-like fashion toward the client's head.

Considerations

The client's low back and hips must always remain firmly in contact with the table to avoid any arching or straining of the client's back.

Hamstrings (Flexed Knee Variation)

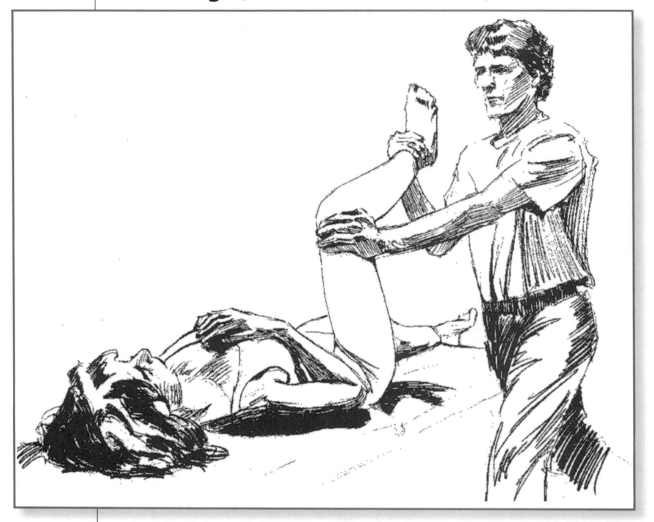

Contract-Relax Procedure

Contraction Phase

Ask your client to flex the knee joint by pulling his/her foot toward the table. Provide resistance with your inside hand.

Stretch Phase

Push the ankle toward the ceiling, stabilizing the leg with your outside hand proximal to the knee; further extend the knee to achieve stretch.

Considerations

The client should not feel the stretch behind the knee joint.

Adductor Group (Straight Leg)

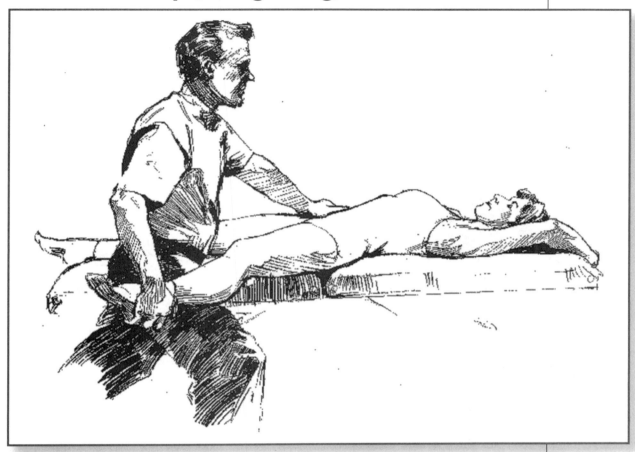

Contract-Relax Procedure

Contraction Phase

Ask your client to press (adduct) the straight leg toward the table. Provide resistance with your own leg or hip.

Stretch Phase

1. Stabilize the client's straight leg just distal to the ankle joint with your outside hand. Be sure the client's foot points toward the ceiling. Stabilize the client's opposite ASIS with your inside hand.

2. Maintaining the leg at the horizontal level of the massage table, abduct the hip in an arc-like fashion outward from the table. Use your body weight, moving forward with the lunge to apply/enhance the stretch.

Note: One variation of this stretch is to allow the knee to flex 90 degrees while supporting just above the knee. This removes gracilis from the stretch and focuses on the adductor group muscles.

Adductor Group (Figure 4)

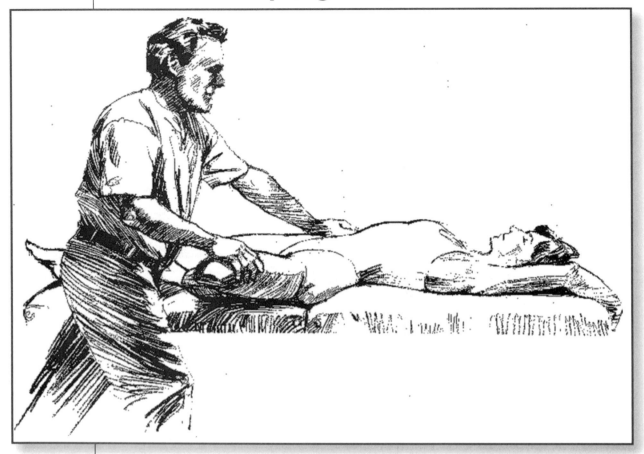

Contract-Relax Procedure

Contraction Phase

Ask your client to press (adduct) the leg (knee) toward the ceiling against your hand, thus engaging the adductor muscles.

Stretch Phase

1. Stabilize the client's leg at the medial aspect of the knee joint with your outside hand; stabilize the client's opposite ASIS with your inside hand.

2. Abduct the hip by pushing the client's knee toward the table.

Quadriceps

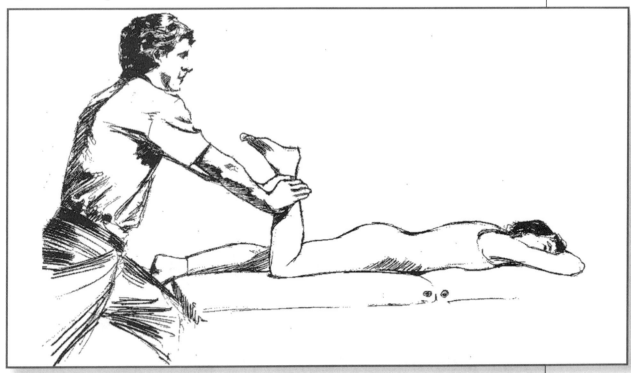

Contract-Relax Procedure

Contraction Phase

1. Bring the client's knee joint to 60°–90° of flexion.

2. Ask your client to press the foot toward the end of the table (extension of the knee). Working from a solid lunge while supporting the client's sacrum/low back, provide resistance with your hand.

   Note: the contraction phase should NEVER take place when the client's knee joint is flexed more than 90°. At such an angle, the tissues of the knee joint and quadriceps tendon are subjected to too much stress. The contraction phase must take place when the knee joint is angled between 60° and 90°.

Stretch Phase

1. Stabilize the client's sacrum with your superior hand, and proximal to the ankle with your inferior hand. Be sure the leg is in a straight line with the client's body.

2. Flex the knee joint by bringing the foot toward the client's hip.

Considerations

Many clients will be flexible enough for the ankle to reach the hip with no stretch, or not feel a stretch in the quadriceps area; if so:

1. Support the sacrum more and/or slightly decompress the sacrum toward the client's feet.

2. Be sure the leg being stretched is in a straight line with the body and not abducted.

3. Have the client tighten the abdominals when applying the stretch (pelvic tilt).

Abductors—Tensor Fascia Latae/Gluteus Medius

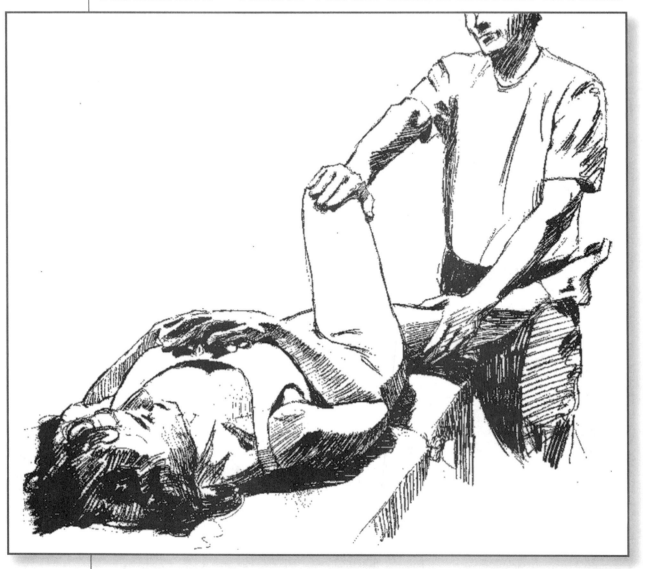

Contract-Relax Procedure

Contraction Phase

Ask your client to press (abduct) the straight leg away from your side of the table. Provide resistance with your leg or hip, or against your supporting hand as in option #2 (see pg. 21).

Stretch Phase

1. Stabilize the straight leg just proximal to the ankle joint with the outside hand, and stabilize the client's other leg at the knee with the inside hand.

2. Maintain the straight leg at the horizontal level of the massage table and adduct the hip in an arc-like fashion toward your side of the table.

Considerations

The client's low back and hips always remain firmly in contact with the table to avoid any arching or straining of the client's back.

Hip Flexors—Rectus Femoris and Iliopsoas

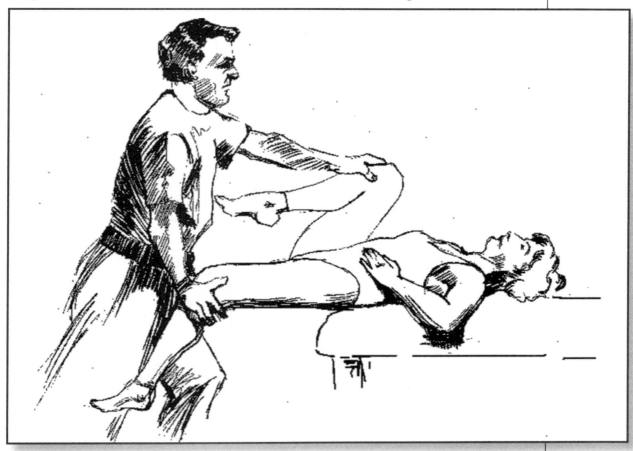

Contract-Relax Procedure

Contraction Phase

Ask your client to press (flex) the leg upward toward the ceiling. Working from a lunge position, provide resistance with your hand. Be sure the client's leg stays in a straight line with his/her hip.

Stretch Phase

1. Stabilize the leg just proximal to the knee joint with your outside hand.
2. Stabilize the other leg at the knee. Be sure to keep the client's low back flat on the table by using this hand to push the client's leg toward their head. This will posteriorly rotate the pelvis.
3. Extend the hip with your outside hand, pushing the leg toward the floor.

Considerations

The client may stabilize the low back by tucking the opposite leg into his/her chest. If the client feels a pinching sensation in the hip, ask him/her to stabilize the leg by grasping behind the upper thigh, just proximal to the knee.

Pectoralis Major

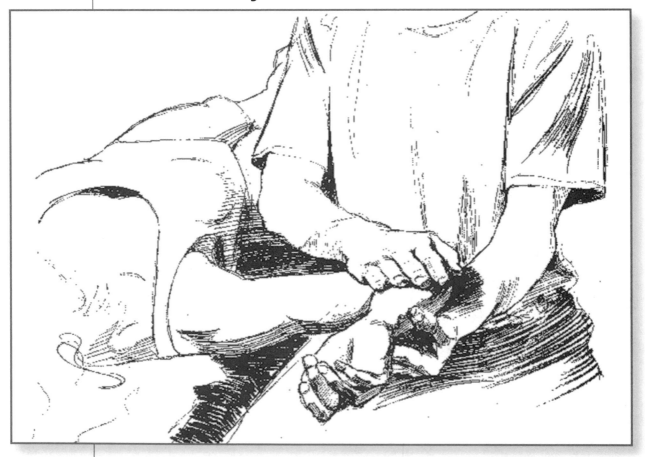

Contract-Relax Procedure

Contraction Phase

1. Bring the arm back to the same horizontal level as the massage table.

2. Ask your client to press (horizontally adduct) the arm toward his/her chest. Provide resistance with your hand just proximal to the elbow. Be sure the client uses his/her elbow to horizontally adduct. The brachial area of the arm should do the work—NOT the forearm.

Stretch Phase

1. Stabilize the forearm from beneath with your outside hand; your inside hand is placed proximal to the client's elbow from above—thus, your two hands face in opposition to each other.

2. Take the client's arm through extension and upward rotation of the scapula. You will be stretching the arm higher over the client's head, while simultaneously pressing the client's arm toward the floor.

Neck Flexion (Supporting Client's Shoulder)

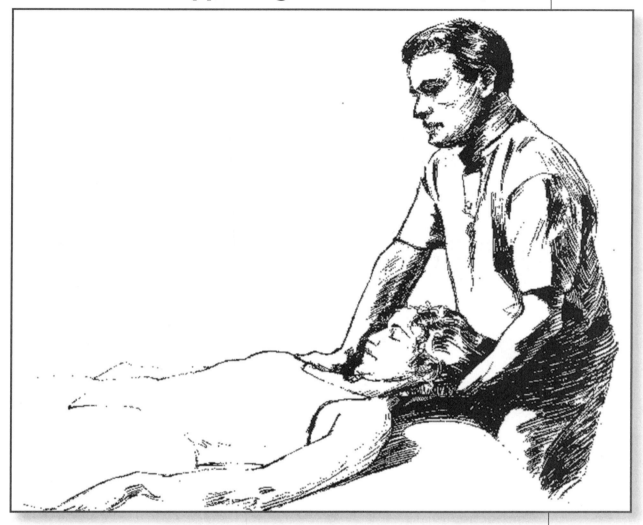

Contract-Relax Procedure

Contraction Phase

1. Bring the head back slightly before providing resistance. Too much flexion could potentially strain the muscles and ligaments.

2. Ask your client to push (extend) the head back toward the table. From a lunge position, provide resistance with your hand.

Stretch Phase

1. Stand at the head of the table in a lunge position.

2. Stabilize one shoulder against the table with your hand on the same side. Stabilize the neck and base of the head (occipital ridge) with your other hand.

3. Flex the neck in an arc-like fashion using your legs to create the movement. Avoid pinning the client's chin to his/her chest.

Neck Flexion (Arms Criss-Cross)

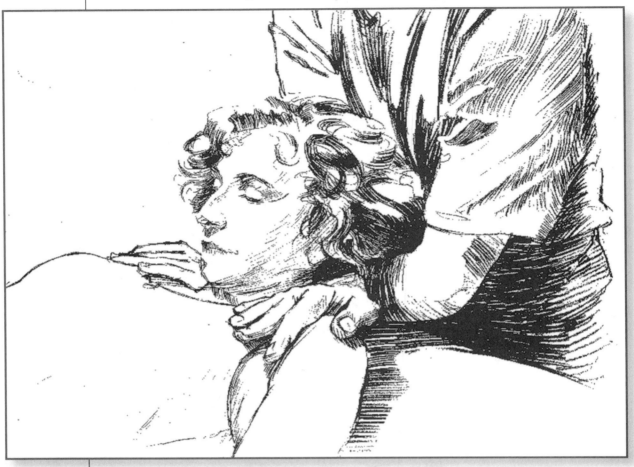

Contract-Relax Procedure

Contraction Phase

1. Bring the client's head back slightly before providing resistance. Too much flexion could strain the muscles and ligaments.

2. Ask the client to push (extend) the head and neck toward the table. Provide resistance with your forearms from a lunge or horse stance position.

Stretch Phase

1. Stabilize the client's shoulders; use as much of your palms as possible. Position yourself low to the table so the client's head rests on your forearms.

2. Flex the client's neck in an arc-like fashion, using your legs to create the movement. Avoid pinning the client's chin to his/her chest.

Neck Lateral Flexion (Arms Criss-Cross)

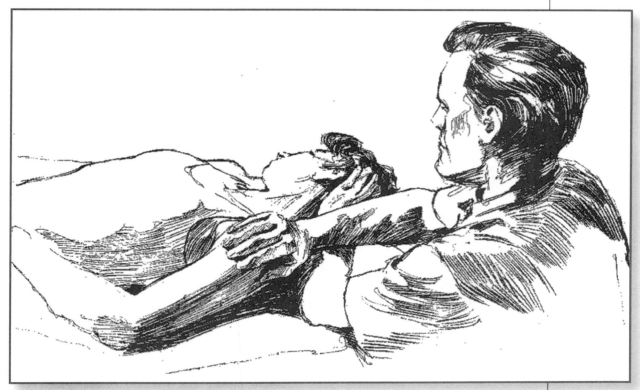

Contract-Relax Procedure

Contraction Phase

1. Bring the head back slightly if the client has great flexibility or range of motion.

2. Ask the client to either press the shoulder upward or attempt to bring the head toward the side being stretched. Provide resistance with both your hands.

Stretch Phase

1. By crossing your arms, stabilize the shoulder with your superior hand and stabilize the base of the head (occipital ridge) with your inferior hand.

2. Laterally flex the neck (with some rotation) in an arc-like fashion, away from the side where you are kneeling.

Latissimus Dorsi/Obliques (Sidelying)

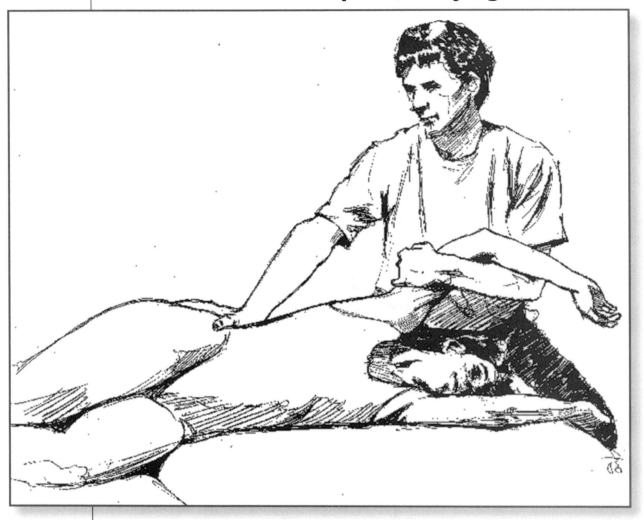

Contract-Relax Procedure

Contraction Phase

1. Ask your client to pull (adduct) their arm downward toward their side. From a lunge position, provide resistance with your hand.

2. Ask your client to simultaneously pull (elevate or hike) the hip up toward the head of the table. Provide resistance with your hand.

Stretch Phase

1. Stand in a lunge position facing the foot of the table.

2. Stabilize the top of the hip by cupping it with your outside/inferior hand.

3. Stabilize the arm with your inside/superior hand by overlapping the your forearm/ elbow with your client's forearm/elbow. Your inside/superior hand should be passing in front of the shoulder.

4. Depress the hip by pushing it down toward the client's feet; simultaneously pull the client's arm overhead.

REFERENCES

Alter, Michael J. (1996) *Science of Flexibility. 2nd edition.* Champaign, IL: Human Kinetics.

Cash, Mel. (1996) *Sport & Remedial Massage Therapy.* London: Ebury Press.

Chaitow, Leon. (1997) *Muscle Energy Techniques.* London: Churchill Livingston.

Fritz, Sandy. (1995) *Mosby's Fundamentals of Therapeutic Massage.* St. Louis: Mosby Lifeline.

Tappan, Frances; Benjamin, Patricia. (1998) *Handbook of Healing Massage Techniques.* Stamford, CT: Appleton and Lange.

RECIPROCAL INHIBITION

Reciprocal Inhibition Theory

The theory for reciprocal inhibition is much less contested than for contract-relax stretching. When a muscle contracts, sensory information is sent to the brain and spinal cord for processing. One of the responses initiated by the spinal cord is to send an inhibitory response to the antagonist muscle. In effect, if the agonist is shortening, the antagonist must lengthen if movement is to occur. The skilled therapist can use this reflex to help stretch the target muscle.

Indications

- Muscle shortness and/or tension
- Postural imbalances
- Neuromuscular re-education
- Muscle spasm

Contraindications

- There are very few contraindications for this technique. As long as the client can safely move a joint and the reciprocal inhibition movements do not cause pain then it can be used.

PROCEDURE FOR RECIPROCAL INHIBITION TECHNIQUE

General Reciprocal Inhibition Protocol

1. Place the client in the correct position for the desired stretch. This is determined by the target muscle, the best ways to stretch it, and any client needs.

2. Determine the client's ROM for the targeted muscle or muscle group through a passive stretch. Feel for the motion barrier, or end-point, of the stretch. This step may also be accomplished by instructing the client to stretch actively.

3. Slowly move the target muscle into a stretched position, feeling for a motion barrier or slight tissue resistance. This should be pain-free and the client may begin to feel a stretch. Do not move too quickly or too far, so as not to stimulate the stretch reflex.

4. Back out ⅓ to ½ from the end point, and instruct the receiver to contract **with the antagonist muscle** against the resistance you provide. Ask the receiver to utilize a maximum of 20–30% of his or her muscle power. You meet the contraction with equal resistance. Hold for approximately 8 seconds.

5. Then, cue the client to relax fully. Ask the client to take a deep, relaxing breath. The therapist should feel the muscle let go and relax fully.

6. After exhalation, move the client to the next motion barrier or next place of slight tissue resistance.

7. Repeat steps 4–6 three to five times. End by taking the client to the next motion barrier and hold for 20–30 seconds. Once in the final stretch position, have the client breathe and focus his/her awareness on the target muscle.

The same tips and precautions apply to reciprocal inhibition as to contract-relax stretching.

Hamstrings (Straight Leg)

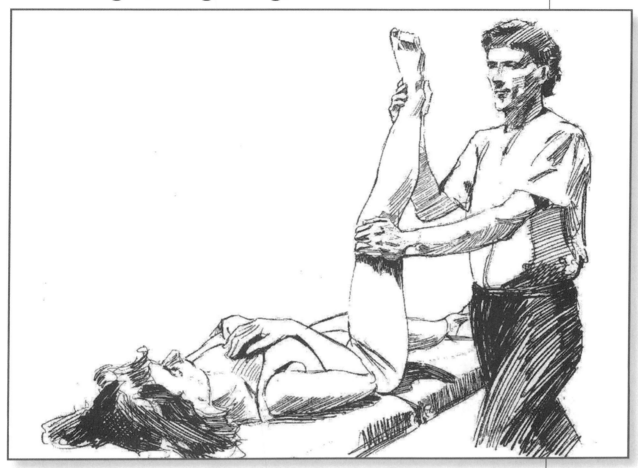

Reciprocal Inhibition Procedure

Contraction Phase

Ask your client to flex his/her hip by pulling the straight leg toward the head, thus activating the iliopsoas muscle. Provide resistance with your outside hand just proximal to the knee joint.

Stretch Phase

1. Stabilize the client's straight leg just proximal to the knee joint with your outside hand; the inside hand is placed behind the client's ankle.
2. Flex the hip in an arc-like fashion toward the client's head.

Considerations

The client's low back and hips always remain firmly in contact with the table to avoid any arching or straining of the client's back.

Hamstrings (Flexed Knee Variation)

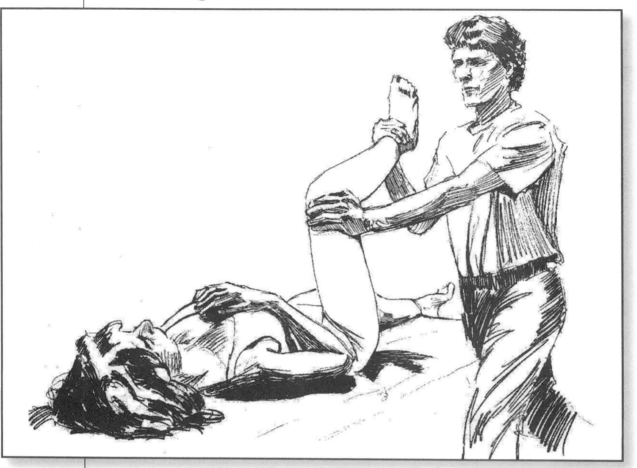

Reciprocal Inhibition Procedure

Contraction Phase

Ask your client to extend the knee joint by pushing the foot toward the ceiling, thus activating the quadriceps muscles. Provide resistance with your inside hand.

Stretch Phase

Push the client's ankle toward the ceiling, stabilizing the leg with your outside hand proximal to the knee; further extend the knee joint to achieve stretch.

Considerations

The client should not feel the stretch behind the knee joint.

Adductor Group (Straight Leg)

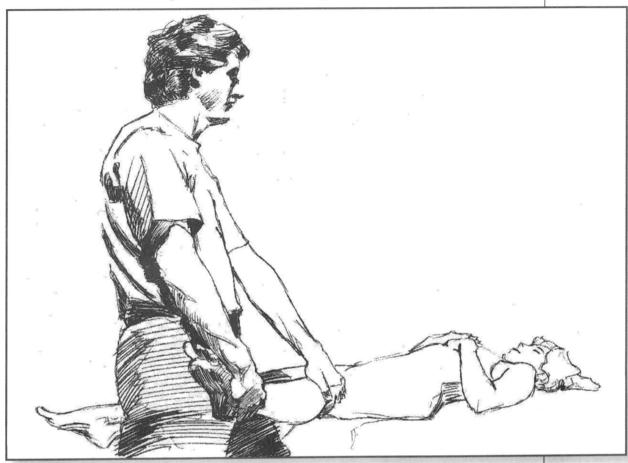

Reciprocal Inhibition Procedure

Contraction Phase

Ask your client to abduct the hip by pushing the straight leg away from the table activating the gluteus medius, gluteus minimus and tensor fascia latae muscles. Provide resistance with your inside hand just proximal to the knee joint.

Stretch Phase

1. Stabilize the client's straight leg just distal to the ankle joint with your outside hand. Be sure the client's foot points toward the ceiling. Stabilize at the client's opposite ASIS with your inside hand.

2. Maintaining the leg at the horizontal level of the massage table, ABduct the hip in an arc-like fashion outward from the table. Use your body weight, moving forward with the lunge to apply or enhance the stretch.

Considerations

The client's low back and hips always remain firmly in contact with the table to avoid any arching or straining of the client's back.

Tensor Fascia Latae/Gluteus Medius (supine position)

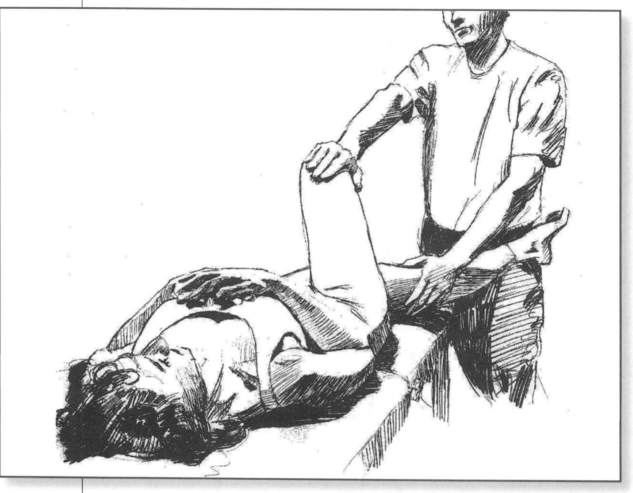

Reciprocal Inhibition Procedure

Contraction Phase

Ask your client to adduct his/her hip by pulling the straight leg away from the table, thus activating the adductor group muscles.

Stretch Phase

1. Stabilize the straight leg just proximal to the ankle joint with your outside hand; stabilize the client's other leg at the knee with your inside hand.

2. Maintain the client's straight leg at the horizontal level of the table; adduct the hip in an arc-like fashion outward from the table.

Considerations

The client's low back and hips always remain firmly in contact with the table to avoid any arching or straining of the client's back.

Gastrocnemius/Soleus
(supine pushing dorsiflexion)

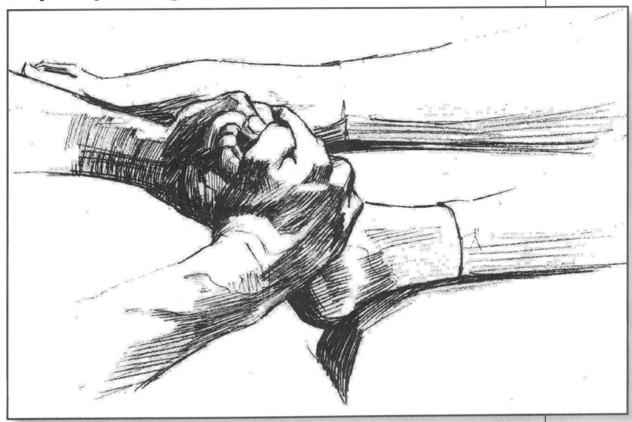

Reciprocal Inhibition Procedure

Contraction Phase

1. Place both your hands (overlapping) on the top of the foot.

2. Ask your client to dorsiflex the ankle by pulling the foot/toes toward his or her body, thus activating the tibialis anterior muscle.

Stretch Phase

1. Stabilize the ankle with your outside hand supporting the lateral malleolus, and your inside hand at the ball of the foot or re-position yourself to passively stretch the calf by pulling into dorsiflexion.

2. Dorsiflex the ankle toward the client's head.

Considerations

Remember, when using Gastrocnemius/Soleus (Supine Pulling Dorsiflexion) you will need to continually reposition yourself with each phase.

Many clients will feel resistance or no stretch in the calf area. If so:

■ Pull with your outside hand, thus stretching the Achilles tendon while simultaneously dorsiflexing the ankle.

■ Have the client sit upright.

Gastrocnemius/Soleus (prone dorsiflexion)

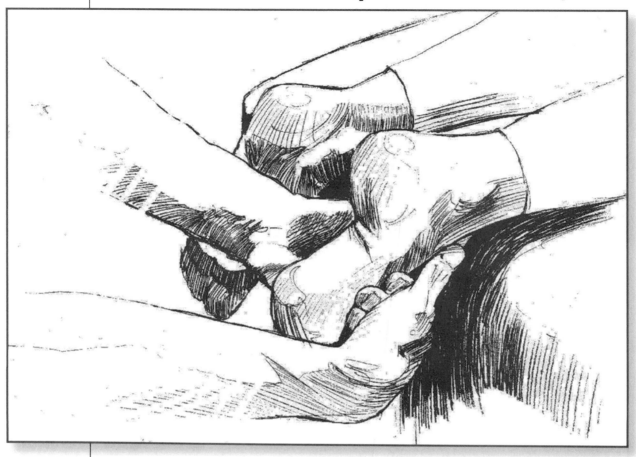

Reciprocal Inhibition Procedure

Contraction Phase

1. Place both your hands (overlapping) on top of the client's foot.
2. Ask the client to dorsiflex the ankle by pulling the foot/toes toward his or her body, thus activating the tibialis anterior muscle.

Stretch Phase

1. Stand in a lunge position facing the head of the table. The ball of the client's foot will be proximal to the knee of your forward leg.
2. Stabilize the calf with your outside hand; your inside hand is placed behind the heel/Achilles tendon.
3. Dorsiflex the ankle toward the table using your weight and leverage from the lunge position. Simultaneously pull the heel/Achilles tendon toward you, thus enhancing the dorsiflexion.

Considerations

If using Gastrocnemius/Soleus–prone dorsiflexion, you will need to continually re-position the hands and stance with each phase.

Many clients will feel resistance or no stretch in the calf area. If so:

- Lean forward into a low lunge position. The client may be receiving more hip elevation than dorsiflexion of the ankle.

- Be sure the client's leg is straight and not tending to bend at the knee joint.

Quadriceps

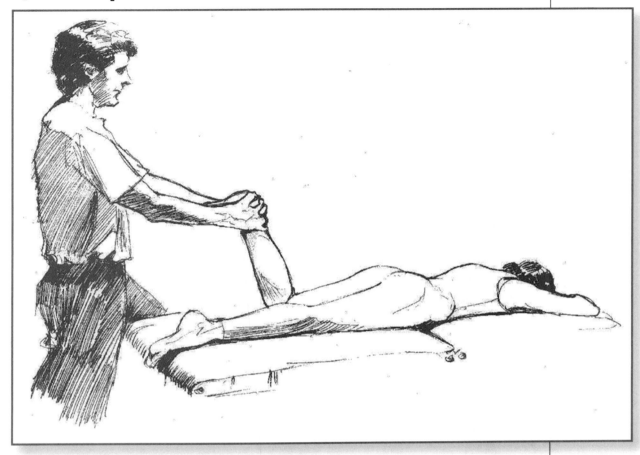

Reciprocal Inhibition Procedure

Contraction Phase

1. Stand in a lunge position facing the head of the table. Bring the client's knee joint to a 90°–130° angle. Place both your hands behind the client's ankle.

2. Ask the client to pull the foot toward his/her hip (flexion of the knee). Working from a lunge position, provide resistance with your hands.

Stretch Phase

1. Stand in a lunge position facing the side of the table at a slight angle.

2. Stabilize the client's sacrum with your superior hand; stabilize proximal to the ankle with your inferior hand. Be sure the leg is in a straight line with the body.

3. Flex the knee joint by bringing the foot toward the client's hip.

Considerations

Many clients will be flexible enough for the ankle to reach the hip without a stretch, or will not feel a stretch in the quadriceps area; if so:

- Support the sacrum more and/or slightly decompress the sacrum toward the client's feet.
- Be sure the leg being stretched is in a straight line with the client's body and not abducted.
- Have the client tighten his or her abdominal muscles as the stretch is applied.

Ilipsoas

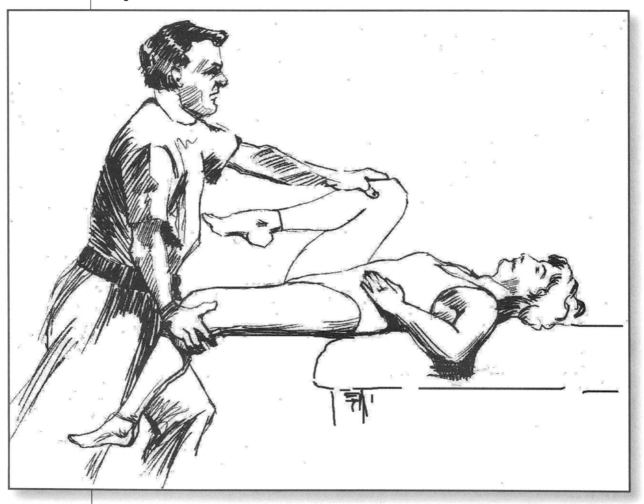

Reciprocal Inhibition Procedure

Contraction Phase

1. Stabilize behind and just proximal to the knee with your outside hand.

2. Ask your client to push (hyperextend) the leg toward the floor, thus activating the hamstring and gluteus maximus muscles.

Stretch Phase

1. Stabilize the leg just proximal to the knee joint with your outside hand.

2. Stabilize the other leg at the knee. Be sure to keep the client's low back flat on the table by using this hand to 'push' the client's leg toward his/her head. This will posteriorly rotate the pelvis.

3. Extend the hip with your outside hand, pushing the leg toward the floor.

Considerations

The client may stabilize the low back by tucking the opposite leg into his/her chest.

If the client feels a pinching sensation in the hip that is tucked, ask the client to stabilize the leg by grasping behind the upper thigh, just proximal to the knee.

Positional Release

POSITIONAL RELEASE

Anyone who is experiencing pain naturally tries to find a position that reduces that unwelcome sensation. This principle of finding a more comfortable position or "position of ease" has been developed into a system of healing and musculoskeletal pain reduction known as **Positional Release.** A therapist can move his/her client into a position that relieves the pain. When the body registers this relief, the normal physiologic mechanisms undo the initial pain-producing pattern and pain relief occurs. The therapist can monitor this change by palpating a tender point, i.e., the key site of pain in the client's body, during the procedure. When the treatment is effective, relief of the tender point occurs. Unlike a trigger point, the tender point produces no referred pain pattern.

Positional Release is a non-invasive and gentle manual therapy technique used to facilitate the body's own healing and self-correction response from painful musculoskeletal conditions. Positional Release consists of the application of a technique wherein the practitioner moves the client's body into a position that reduces the strain and pain in a hypertonic muscle. This allows the nervous system to reset and normalize the muscle, thereby reducing the pain.

Tender Point (TeP)

- Small zone of tense and exquisitely tender myofascial tissue.
- May or may not be palpable as a specific nodule or band.
- Hypersensitive to mechanical pressure.
- Does not produce referred pain pattern. The client is often not aware of it until compressed.
- Neuromuscular origin.
- Tender points indicate stress and strain in that muscle causing a hypersensitive (facilitated) spinal segment.
- Commonly occur at muscle attachments (musculotendinous junctions) and are often found in overly-contracted stressed muscles.
- Restricts movement and is resistant to stretch/lengthening until reflexive contraction is relieved.
- Key indicator for confirming a TeP is the jump response (client tends to flinch and/or pull away from pressure being applied).
- How it develops:
  1. Muscle is held in a shortened position for a long time, then the muscle suddenly lengthens.
  2. Stretch reflex contraction will occur even though the muscle is not being stretched.
  3. Sets up a false stretch reflex signal which makes the muscle spindle hypersensitive to sudden lengthening.
  4. Protective spasm is the end result.

Positional Release techniques can be used with nearly any population but is very commonly used with those in acute or chronic pain. Because it is a less invasive approach, it can be very beneficially used with:

- Fibromyalgia sufferers
- Osteoarthritis cases
- Infants
- The elderly
- Pregnant women
- Post-operative patients (for pain)
- Respiratory difficulties

Benefits

Many benefits can be derived from the use of positional release techniques:

- Decreased muscular hypertonicity and neuromuscular hyper-irritability
- Decreased spasms/muscle guarding
- Decreased pain associated with tender points
- Increased functional mobility for joints
- Improved posture

Positional Release Procedure

1. Locate and palpate the appropriate tender point.
2. Move the client's body into the "position of ease."
3. Hold the position for a minimum of 90 seconds.
4. Gently move back to neutral or starting position.
5. Reassess the tender point.
6. Repeat steps 1–5 until normalization occurs.

POSITIONAL RELEASE METHODOLOGY

It is important to remember that positional release techniques can be used in many circumstances: alleviating tender points, working with strain and injury, or any excess muscle tension. The procedure described here utilizes tender points for assessment and evaluation of effectiveness.

1. **Locate and palpate the appropriate tender point.** Apply brief firm pressure to confirm the tender point. You will know you are on the tender point if the tissue is more tender than the surrounding area (but does not refer), or you may notice a jump sign, a sudden jerking motion, grasping of the therapist's hand, facial grimace, or vocal expletive. Once it has been confirmed, slowly ease up on your pressure so you can gently monitor the point.

2. **Move the client's body into the "position of ease."** This involves the therapist passively shortening the muscle around the tender point, which generally brings the joint into a flexed position (the origin and insertion coming closer together). At the position of ease, the discomfort will be decreased by 70% or so. You will also feel the tissues slacken or let go. If the discomfort does not decrease by 70%, you will need to fine-tune the position by introducing a very small degree of additional movement in order to find the position of maximum ease. Additional ease can often be achieved by asking the client to evaluate which phase of the breathing cycle reduces pain, and then having the client hold that state as comfortably as he/she can. The position of ease is unique for each client and each area.

3. **Hold the position for a minimum of 90 seconds.** Jones found that 90 seconds seemed to give the best results. During this time you should occasionally palpate the tender point with brief firm pressure to monitor how the release is progressing. As you progress in your positional release skills, your monitoring may occur less frequently.

4. **Gently move back to neutral or starting position.** It is important that this is done slowly, so as not to activate protective spindle reflexes.

5. **Reassess the tender point.** Apply brief firm pressure into the tender point to confirm that it is no longer sensitive.

TeP Guidelines

(from *Therapeutic Massage in Athletics,* Archer)

- Treat the most sensitive TeP first.
- Treat proximal to distal.
- Evaluate and treat larger joints and muscles before smaller ones.
- When a cluster of points occurs, treat the center of the cluster.
- When multiple TeP's occur in a row, treat the middle point first.

COMMON AREAS TO FIND TENDER POINTS

While you can utilize positional release anywhere, listed below are 3 common areas you can practice.

1. Upper Trapezius

Tender points are located approximately centrally in the posterior or anterior fibers.

Client is supine with the head rotated and laterally flexed toward the side being treated while the therapist uses the positioning of the ipsilateral (same side) arm to reduce reported tender point pain at least 70%. The position commonly used is one that involves shoulder abduction, external rotation and slight shoulder flexion.

2. Pectoralis Major

Tender points are located on the muscle's lateral border close to the anterior axillary line.

Client is supine. Therapist moves the ipsilateral arm into flexion and adduction (arm goes across the chest). Fine-tuning involves changing the degree of flexion and adduction. You may add traction if this doesn't increase tenderness.

3. Piriformis

Tender points are located somewhere in the belly of the muscle.

Client is prone. Bring the knee into flexion and extend the hip slightly. You can bring your knee under the thigh for support. Then use external rotation of the hip to find the position of ease.

Trigger Points

TRIGGER POINTS

Trigger Points can develop in muscles as a result of trauma, overuse, poor posture, etc. They cause referred pain and discomfort, limit ROM and decrease a muscle's efficiency. Considering these causes and symptoms, we can see how common this problem can be. Probably most working people, athletes and physically active people have had an activation of a trigger point at one time or another, hence the referred pain and discomfort that it produces. We can see, for this reason, why it is vital that a massage therapist be skilled in the use of Trigger Point Therapy.

Definition

A trigger point is defined by Travell and Simons as "a focus of hyperirritability in a tissue that, when compressed, is locally tender and, if sufficiently hypersensitive, gives rise to referred pain and tenderness, and sometimes to referred autonomic phenomena and distortion of proprioception."

Trigger points develop as a result of changes in normal soft tissue starting with excess muscle tension (hypertonicity), retained metabolic waste and relative ischemia, which, if they persist, disturb the functioning of the muscle fibers.

This condition causes an increase in excitation to the spinal cord and facilitation of the associated spinal segment. The reflex arc becomes hypersensitive, the muscle is unable to relax, and an active trigger point results. The excitation can spill over to adjacent segments, associated muscles can tighten up, and further symptoms may develop.

Types of Trigger Points

- **Active:** Active trigger points are always tender, prevent full lengthening, weaken the muscle, and produce a referred pain pattern. They may be:

  - **Primary:** Trigger points activated by acute or chronic overload of a muscle. Or, they may be:

  - **Secondary:** Trigger points that become active because of their reaction to a muscle containing a primary trigger point. Or,

  - **Satellite:** Trigger points that become active because the muscle is in a zone of reference from another muscle's trigger point.

- **Latent:** Trigger points that are painful only when pressed but produce no referred pain pattern.

Associated Trigger Points

- When deactivating trigger points in an involved muscle, one must be aware of trigger points that may develop secondarily in muscles that work closely with its synergists and antagonists.

Referral Patterns

Trigger points may elicit pain on being pressed or may be tender and radiate pain without pressure. Pressing on an active trigger point usually intensifies pain in the reference zone of the trigger point.

Sensory, motor, and autonomic phenomena may be 'triggered' by active trigger points. These include pain, tenderness, increased motor unit activity (spasm), vasoconstriction (blanching), coldness, sweating, pilomotor response, vasodilation, and hypersecretion. These effects often occur at a distance from the trigger point, but within the general area to which a specific trigger point refers pain (Travell and Simons, 1992, p.5).

Trigger Point (TrPt)

- Hyperirritable nodule within skeletal muscle giving rise to extreme pain with only moderate compression.

- Palpable taut band.

- Development believed to be dysfunction at synapse between motor neuron and muscle fiber (neuromuscular junction).

- Characteristic referred pain pattern into surrounding tissues with pressure.
- The muscle housing the TrPt is hypersensitive to stretch.
- Visual or tactile local twitch response.
- Altered sensation in the muscle housing the TrPt.

Resources

Tappan and Benjamin, (1998) *Tappan's Handbook of Healing Massage Techniques,* Simon & Schuster Company.

CAUSES OF TRIGGER POINTS

Precipitating factors that can contribute to TrP activation or development.

1. **Increased Mechanical Strain**

   ■ Overuse

   ■ Repetition

   ■ Misuse

2. **Ischemia**

   ■ Muscle tension can restrict arterial flow.

3. **Trauma**

   ■ Local inflammatory response at acute injury sites.

   ■ Chemicals released stimulate nociceptors that produce the sensation of pain.

   ■ Leads to pain-spasm-pain cycle and more spasms.

4. **Disuse or Prolonged Immobility**

   ■ Decreased circulation.

5. **Mental/Emotional Distress**

   ■ Prolonged Sympathetic Nervous System arousal can lead to TrP activation.

Pathophysiology of a TrPt

When we overuse, misuse, disuse or abuse, the result is TrPt development. It is the dysfunction of muscle tone, strength, flexibility, pain, and vasoconstriction.

TRIGGER POINT ASSESSMENT & TREATMENT

Below is a series of important steps that, when performed correctly, will give the best results in releasing a trigger point and thereby reduce pain.

1. Warm the Tissues

In order to work deeper into the tissues and to release the TrP, the massage therapist must first prepare the tissues. This includes improving circulation, warming the connective tissue ground substance, and bringing the client into a parasympathetic mode which puts the client into a relaxed state.

Techniques that effectively warm the tissues are compression, effleurage and kneading. Gentle muscle stripping may also be useful.

2. Location & Identification of Trigger Points

- Once the tissues have been warmed and the client is relaxed, it is easier to focus on the exact nodule where the TrP is located. The client is also in a state that makes him/her more receptive to the treatment.
- Locate the area of discomfort and palpate the muscle.
- Find the taut band within the muscle using moderate pressure and work sensitively; excess pressure can irritate the TrP.
- Find the nodule within the taut band; the TrP is within the nodule.
- Check with the client that you have the spot; it will be exquisitely tender.
- Apply digital compression on the TrP.
- A local twitch response may occur.
- If the referred pain pattern is reproduced, this confirms the presence of a trigger point.
- Only palpate the TrP's that you will be able to treat in that session.
- Palpation of a trigger point can aggravate the referred pain pattern unless you release it.

3. Focal Compression

- This technique has been shown to effectively release TrP's.
- **Methods**
  - Use your thumb, fingers or elbow
  - Apply perpendicular to tissue, or
  - Use a controlled pincer grasp of the muscle
- **Amount of Pressure**
  - Maintain communication with the client regarding pressure, TrPt location and effectiveness of the work
  - Gradually sink into the tissues with enough pressure to create discomfort within the client's level of tolerance (e.g., 4–6 on a 1 to 10 discomfort scale; or mild to moderate discomfort)
  - Keep the pressure steady
  - Pressure can be increased as the release occurs
  - Decrease pressure if the tissue tenses; excessive pressure will cause the client to tense up and not be able to release
- **Application of Pressure**
  - Depends on the client's response to your treatment, the amount of pressure, and the condition of the tissues. In some cases, you may hold the pressure for a short period of time or longer, until the release occurs.
  - If the level of discomfort is decreasing, continue to hold the point until the discomfort has leveled off (no more change) or has disappeared, then slowly release the pressure.

- If the discomfort has increased or not changed, slowly release the pressure, then apply techniques to promote circulation (e.g. friction, gliding, kneading, lifting strokes, etc.), then repeat focal compression.
- If there is no change, there may be perpetuating factors, or the trigger point is not ready to release.
- Spend no more than 15 minutes treating trigger points in a specific area.

4. Local Circulatory Techniques

- Once the trigger point is released, it is important to flush metabolic byproducts out of the tissues and to allow fresh oxygenated blood to perfuse the tissues, using techniques such as effleurage, cross-fiber friction or kneading

5. Lengthening/Stretching

- Stretch is an essential component of trigger point therapy. Incomplete restoration of normal muscle length and tone usually means incomplete relief of pain. Certain massage techniques also lengthen the muscle: repetitive muscle stripping, myofascial techniques, and the slow gliding stretch of the muscle called "muscle lengthening."
- Should generally be applied after the above techniques
- Helps to normalize the neuromuscular setting

6. Reassessment

- After completing the above steps, the TrPt and the client's condition should be reassessed. This includes evaluating the referral pain pattern, the quality of the tissues, and how the client feels.
- If you have achieved the desired results, the session is complete, or this portion of your session is finished.
- If you have not achieved the desired results, repeat the treatment procedure or some portion of it until you achieve the desired results.
- If Trigger Point Therapy is not decreasing the discomfort level, see the section below.

- **Other Techniques**
  - Once the therapist has the skills for working with trigger points, he/she can use other techniques besides focal compression to get the same results.
  - Cross-fiber (transverse) friction and kneading may also be effective.
  - Proprioceptive techniques and positional release may also work.

TRIGGER POINT THERAPY PROCEDURE

1. **Apply ischemic compression.** Locate the area of discomfort and gradually apply specific digital compression with moderate pressure.

2. **Confirm the level of discomfort.** Get verbal confirmation that you are on the spot and ask about the degree of discomfort being experienced. You can use a rating scale from 1–10 where 1 equals almost no discomfort and 10 equals unbearable discomfort. This procedure seems to be most effective when the level of discomfort is moderate or at a level of 5–6 on the 1–10 scale as described above. However, the trigger point procedure can be performed at other levels of discomfort. Caution: too much discomfort will create bracing or armoring and will stimulate the nervous system more. You can also inquire about any referred phenomena. Referred sensation can lend important clues about the severity of the condition.

3. **Hold the Trigger Point for 90 seconds.** Once you have confirmed the level of discomfort, hold the point with steady pressure for approximately 90 seconds. As you get started, be certain not to vary your pressure. Any variance will once again stimulate the nervous system. As the point starts to release, gradually increase your pressure by melting into the tissue.

4. **Check in again—is there any change?** While still applying compression, after 30 seconds, check in again. Ask if there has been any change in the primary site or in the referral area. The client's response to this question will determine what your next step will be.

    a. The referral is gone . . . gradually release the point.

    b. If the discomfort is still releasing, continue to hold the point until the discomfort has leveled off (no more change) or has disappeared.

    c. If the discomfort has either increased or not changed, the TrPt is not ready to release.

5. **Slowly release the point.**

6. After releasing the point, **apply techniques to promote circulation**—like friction, effleurage, or pétrissage, and apply a light stretch to the area for 15–30 seconds to further encourage release of the contraction knot.

7. **Repeat.** You will need to return to the same point to apply the above progression repeatedly. Assess to see if the initial level of discomfort has decreased since the previous application.

8. **Follow up with lengthening and stretch immediately or at the end of the session.**

9. Encourage the client to drink water to rehydrate tissue and restore proper lubrication and spacing between collagen and muscle fibers.

10. Perpetuating factors causing TrPts must be understood by the client and eliminated or reduced.

REASONS FOR WHICH THE TRIGGER POINT TREATMENT IS NOT DECREASING COMFORT

There may be times when the application of Trigger Point Therapy is not immediately effective, as indicated by the persistence, or possible increase, of the client's discomfort level. There are many potential explanations for this occurrence:

1. You are not on the correct spot. The sensitive spot is not the primary cause of pain. It is a symptom of the problem. Discomfort may be experienced even though you may not be on its source. Assess the nearby area to see if the center of the sensitivity is there. You may need to search other muscles or parts of the same muscle.

2. You may be on a satellite TrPt and not on the primary TrPt.

3. You may simply need to change your angle of engagement; e.g., come in at the side of the muscle instead of the top, or vice versa.

4. You have not warmed sufficiently. Not enough warming leaves the tissue unprepared for change.

5. You released pressure rather than sustaining pressure.

6. You are using too much pressure. Too much pressure is counterproductive and may result in stimulating the reflex arc. Initially pressing too hard causes involuntary tensing by the client.

7. You are using too little pressure. Too little pressure will not override the prevailing state of the nervous system and will not cause any change.

8. The client may have an underlying condition (e.g., muscle strain, tendonitis, bursitis, intervertebral lesion, etc).

9. The client may have perpetuating factors that continue to make the TrPt hyperirritable. If, after a number of successful treatments, the trigger point and its symptoms have a tendency of returning and persisting, there may be a perpetuating factor. If this is the case, the client should attempt to resolve this in order to support the trigger point therapy and to achieve permanent relief of symptoms.

   - **Mechanical:** postural misalignments, gait abnormalities, immobilization, work stress, ill-fitting attire or shoes, or ergonomically dysfunctional furniture

   - **Reflexive:** joint dysfunction, visceral dysfunction, vasoconstriction, or a facilitated nerve segment

   - **Systemic:** illness, chronic infection, nutritional deficiencies or psychological factors

10. The body tissue is simply not ready to change or is too irritable. Leave the area for a while and then return. Sometimes a little extra time is necessary for the increased circulation to have its effect.

HEAT VS. COLD FOR TRIGGER POINT THERAPY

The intent of Trigger Point Therapy is to override the hyper-facilitated reflex arc, giving the muscle an opportunity to relax, seek homeostasis and proper tonus. The therapist is utilizing sustained compression with moderate pressure in combination with circulatory techniques. When applied appropriately, Trigger Point Therapy does not elicit the body's inflammatory response. The use of heat (preferably moist) will aid circulation and relax the ischemic band of tissue that is causing the hyperirritable spot.

In the case of using direct friction variations, or other techniques, to break up a fibrotic matrix where chronic inflammation is present, the intent is to use the body's own inflammatory response to aid the healing process. In these circumstances of purposeful activation of inflammatory response, as with any acute inflammation, the application of cold (ice) is indicated.

Other uses of friction, such as warming, loosening, and tissue broadening, do not elicit the body's inflammatory response. Therefore, integrating friction with trigger point procedures does not automatically mean that cold must be used. When indicating whether a client should use heat or cold after a massage, the therapist must ask whether or not inflammation has been induced. Intuition and experience will help guide the therapist as to the appropriate response.

MASSAGE TREATMENT PROTOCOL FOR TRIGGER POINT THERAPY

History

- Description of pain, location, intensity, duration
- Activation, determine if pain was caused by acute or chronic overload
- What makes it better or worse?
- How does it feel right now?
- Have you sought medical attention for this problem?

Testing

- Check range of motion to help determine which muscles are affected
- Determine which movements are limited
- Is there pain when certain muscles are stretched?

Palpation (to determine the exact location of the trigger point)

- Transverse friction, circular friction, pincer compression, flat palpation

Trigger Point Approach (hands-on treatment)

- Exact site to include: angle, direction of engagement, correct body position of client, correct body position of therapist
- Sustained ischemic pressure (8–12 seconds approximately)
- Repeat sustained pressure (2–4 times) while integrating other loosening techniques for the specific band or fiber where the trigger point is located
- Moist heat (before or after stretch)
- Stretch involving the muscle band or muscle group (passive stretch, active assisted stretch variations)
- Active range of motion of involved muscles

Corrective Actions (eliminating perpetuating factors and minimizing predisposing factors)

- Rearrange the work place
- Develop proper sitting, standing, lifting and sleeping postures
- Avoid stress overload of involved muscles
- Keep affected muscles warm
- Exercise to increase the stress tolerance of involved muscles

Home Treatment (self-care)

- Ischemic compression
- Moist heat or hot shower
- Stretch and active range of motion of affected muscles
- Strengthen and stretch exercises, i.e., balance boards, gymnastic balls, wall stabilization exercise, tennis ball therapy

Sports Massage

SPORTS MASSAGE INTRODUCTION

Over the past few decades there have been tremendous strides in the growth and advancement of sports science. Sports science includes the study of physiology, health, exercise, training, nutrition, hydration, injury, rehabilitation, and psychology in relation to athletic and competitive performance. For the most part, advances in sports science have been responsible for the ever-increasing abilities and levels of performance of our athletes today. In addition, the knowledge and techniques gained through sports science have begun to have a large impact on medicine and health care as a whole, especially in the areas of rehabilitation and physical therapy.

Concurrent with this growth has been the wider recognition and acceptance of ongoing massage therapy as a means of supporting athletic performance, training, and recovery. Nearly all professional sports teams now provide massage therapy for their athletes. Massage has been available at all of the Olympics in recent history, and many national and collegiate teams employ massage therapists.

Definition

Sports Massage is a rapidly developing specialty within the field of massage therapy. More and more athletes are recognizing that massage therapy is not only a useful adjunct to their training but can give them a competitive edge. Sports Massage should not be considered an entirely different approach to massage because it does not necessarily define a new or different type of massage technique. Sports Massage therapists merely take the tools and techniques of Western massage therapy and adapt them for this specific population.

Benjamin and Lamp (*Understanding Sports Massage,* 1996) define Sports Massage as "the science and art of applying massage and related techniques to ensure the health and well-being of the athlete and to enhance athletic performance." Simply put, Sports Massage is massage therapy applied in the context of athletic training and competition to meet the specific goals and needs of the athlete. That said, all massage therapists benefit from learning the skills and approaches of sports massage. Many of our 'nonathlete' clients, in work or play, engage in many sport-like activities and can benefit from the knowledge and approaches of Sports Massage. You might think of an executive assistant as a 'typing athlete,' someone with a 'green thumb' as a 'gardening athlete,' or a massage therapist as a 'massage athlete.' Although not competitive, these people have some of the same needs and potential for injury as someone training for competition. Your introduction to the basic concepts and approaches of Sports Massage is provided so that you can apply them when working with athletes and non-athletes alike. It is not intended to certify the student as a Sports Massage Therapist.

The type of massage given to an athlete varies according to these factors:

- Timing—when the massage is performed: before an event, during an event, after an event, or during training.

- Setting or location of the massage

- Sport—which body areas are biomechanically stressed

- Status of tissue—healthy, injured or overtrained

- Athlete's medical history

PRINCIPLES OF SPORTS MASSAGE

There have historically been many definitions of (and disagreements about) the scope of Sports Massage. Early definitions limited its scope to massage applied immediately before or after an event. Modern definitions have been expanded to include ongoing work with an athlete in conjunction with his or her training.

Sports Massage can be divided into two primary categories. These categories are related to the venue in which massage is applied. Within these categories are subcategories which are distinguished by intent, set of goals, and application.

1. **Event Massage,** which includes:

   ■ Pre-event massage

   ■ Inter- or intra-event massage

   ■ Post-event massage

2. **Training Massage,** which includes:

   ■ Recovery massage

   ■ Maintenance massage

   ■ Treatment massage

The distinguishing characteristics of these categories (and subcategories) will be discussed more thoroughly later in this manual. However, all forms of Sports Massage do share some common goals.

Goals of Sports Massage

The specific goals of Sports Massage are really derived from the goals of the athlete. An athlete desires to engage in training that will gradually improve his/her skills and performance in order to perform well in competition. In order to achieve his or her goals, the athlete, with the assistance of the massage therapist, needs to:

1. Be able to participate in high-quality training and competition.

2. Recover from training exercises and competition quickly (especially those that push the athlete's capabilities) in order to more quickly return to high level training.

3. Prevent the onset of injuries.

4. If injuries develop, recover or rehabilitate from those injuries as quickly as possible.

Some athletic training can be viewed as the controlled application of 'trauma' to the body. By pushing their bodies to the limits of performance, athletes are slightly traumatizing the body so that the body responds by making itself stronger, faster, and more enduring. The body does this by:

1. Adding more cells in stressed tissues such as tendons and ligaments.

2. Making the cells larger in tissues such as muscle.

3. Building more venous and arterial capillaries, thus providing more and better nutrition and oxygenation to the tissues.

4. Increasing the body's ability to convert fuel into energy and replenish its energy stores quickly.

The role of the sports massage therapist is to support the goals of the athlete and to assist the athlete's body in responding appropriately to the stresses placed upon it. This role is performed in cooperation with the athlete, trainer, coach, nutritionist, or any other professional partnering to help the athlete excel.

BENEFITS OF SPORTS MASSAGE

The direct effects of Sports Massage are no different than those of most other types of massage therapy. Again, the massage techniques are just applied in a way that specifically benefits the needs of the athlete. Let's look more closely at how the benefits of Sports Massage relate to the needs and goals of the athlete.

Supports High-Quality Training and Competition

- Maintains optimal health of soft tissues. Enhanced circulatory effect, additional blood and lymph flow, helps soft tissues maintain optimal condition.

- Promotes a positive mental attitude.

- Promotes relaxation, helps to stimulate and invigorate, and can be a positive part of the athlete's ritual. Massage, and the massage therapist, can be an important emotional support during training.

- Reduces pain. Decreased pain improves the athlete's ability to perform at a high level. Pain is a definite performance inhibitor.

- Prepares the tissues for use. Massage readies the tissues, assisting in their attainment of an optimal state prior to training or competition.

Reduces Recovery Time For Quicker Return To Training and Competition

- Speeds replenishment of depleted energy stores in the muscles.

- Increases the availability of nutrient-rich blood and promotes phagocytosis to speed healing.

- Promotes the elimination of built-up metabolites in the tissues that result from muscular training.

- Reduces delayed onset muscle soreness, enabling the athlete to train and perform more consistently at a higher level.

- Reduces cramping, spasm, and voluntary/involuntary splinting, thus promoting a complete recovery and improved muscle balance.

Prevents the Onset of Injuries

- Assessment helps identify and subsequently treat potential injuries before they fully develop and become disabling.

- Reduces hypertonicity of muscles, creating improved tone, and relaxation; promotes overall muscle balance.

- Optimizes range of motion and flexibility—a key component to reducing the potential for injury.

- Reduces the inflammatory processes that can lead to secondary injury.

- Reduces the formation of adhesions and scar tissue, allowing for freer movement, re-established functioning, range of motion, and promotion of muscle balance.

- Increases body awareness, thus helping the athlete to know when they are 'over-training,' especially if a problem is developing.

Recover or Rehabilitate From Injuries as Quickly as Possible

- Immediate ice application (and Rest, Ice, Compression and Elevation [RICE]) can reduce acute inflammation to promote quicker healing.

- The use of massage and cryostretch can help relieve mild muscle spasms.

Direct treatment of injuries (scar tissue, muscle imbalance, trigger points, etc.) aids in a more rapid and complete recovery from an injury, thus reducing the likelihood of chronic problems and further, or repeated, injury.

PRE-EVENT MASSAGE

Purpose

For an athlete, the warm-up is an integral part of an event or workout. It is very important to create a state of readiness in the muscles and tissues by stimulating circulation and bringing in a fresh, abundant supply of blood ready to supply the tissues once exercise begins. Tendons, ligaments, muscle fibers, and fascial tissues need to be freed and lubricated so that tissues can move and contract without hindrance. Hypertonic muscles should be relaxed and range of motion optimized. This not only enhances performance but also helps prevent injuries. Mental preparation is also important and can include relaxation, focused concentration, centering, and visualization.

Pre-event massage is given as an adjunct—not a substitute—to the athlete's actual physical warm-up. It has important physiological and psychological benefits. It helps the muscles to work longer and more efficiently by increasing circulation, reducing muscle tension, and increasing the flexibility of tight muscle groups. It can enhance the athlete's general state of wellbeing, which will help him/her create an optimal state for performance.

Timing

There are many factors that influence the optimal timing for administering a pre-event massage. In many cases, 15–90 minutes before the event may be best. However, this is dependent on the event itself, the condition of the athlete, and the practicality of providing the massage, especially when working with a number of athletes. Another important factor is the massage therapist's familiarity with a particular athlete, that athlete's past experience, and how that athlete responds to massage. The athlete's response to massage depends very much on how frequently they've received it before, as such therapy is a physiological learning experience.

PRE-EVENT MASSAGE: OVERVIEW

Description—Pre-Event Massage Is:

- Non-specific—focus is on major muscle groups
- Not deep—deep techniques that require recovery are contraindicated
- Warming—focus is on increasing circulation and loosening tissues
- Short in duration—15–20 minutes maximum up to two hours prior to the event
- Event-specific—emphasis is on muscles to be used for the particular event, especially hypertonic areas
- Invigorating—should be up-tempo, rhythmic pace to relax and stimulate; should not put athlete 'to sleep' or allow the athlete to 'zone out'
- Painless—no pain should be experienced (deep, digital pressure is contraindicated)
- Intentional—the intent is to prepare the athlete for competition, not to make changes in his or her body

Goals of Pre-Event Massage

- Warm up athlete's tissues—especially in areas stressed by the specific event
- Increase circulation to the tissues
- Lubricate joints
- Lubricate and free fascial structures
- Relax hypertonic muscles
- Create a state of relaxed preparedness

TECHNIQUES

Most of the massage techniques you have learned so far can be utilized in a Pre-event Sports Massage. Gliding techniques are not used because they necessitate the use of a lubricant and the athlete is dressed in a pre-event setting. Also, lubricants on the skin will alter the athlete's temperature regulation systems, and are therefore best avoided.

Although many techniques can be utilized in pre-event work, the massage itself is characteristically short in duration. Therefore, it is usually best to use techniques that will most efficiently and effectively achieve the goals of the massage, such as:

- **Compression Variations**—Compression techniques, when applied appropriately, can very quickly relax and warm large muscle groups. All three variations (simple, rhythmic, and fiber-spreading) can be utilized. Fiber-spreading may be particularly useful in broadening and freeing muscle fibers and fascial tissues.

- **Pétrissage**—Pétrissage is a great warming stroke that increases local circulation and lifts tissues from the underlying structures. Compression and pétrissage working together act like a mechanical pump for pushing fluids out and bringing fresh blood into the tissues.

- **Generalized Friction Techniques**—Using the palm of the hand to apply broader friction strokes can really warm tissues. General fingertip friction (transverse and/or circular) to areas of tendons and ligaments will unstick fibrotic tissues and help lubricate these normally ischemic areas.

- **Jostling & Passive Movement Techniques**—In short duration, jostling stimulates proprioceptors and is invigorating to the muscles. Passive movement is great for lubricating synovial joints. Both techniques have great psychological benefits by creating a sense of freedom in movement.

- **Movement Techniques**—Movement is great for lubricating synovial joints and for further freeing of the tissues. This has great psychological benefits by creating a sense of freedom.

- **Percussion**—In short duration, percussion can be invigorating for the athlete and get him/her ready for action.

- **Gentle Stretching**—The intent of stretching in pre-event massage is not to create new expanses in range of motion. Stretching techniques in pre-event work are used only to help return hypertonic tissue to normal length and as a warming technique. However, the guidelines of stretching must still be followed. Muscles should be warmed prior to attempting a stretch.

CONTRAINDICATIONS/CAUTIONS

All the normal contraindications are to be respected in a pre-event massage. There are also a few specific cautions to be considered:

- **No specific, deep, or clinical treatment oriented massage.** Massage that creates pain, specific trauma, or the need for recovery are inappropriate when an athlete is going to be stressing the tissues. Creating pain or trauma can have a very negative effect on performance and the athlete's mindset.

- **Do not over-stretch.** Not only is there the potential for creating injury but, you will be resetting proprioception. In a sport that necessitates precision (e.g., pitching a baseball, swinging a golf club, etc.), changing a person's proprioception can significantly affect his/her ability to perform accurately.

- **No ice application.** Although ice applied for longer periods increases circulation, within the short time frame of a pre-event massage, the application of ice would only serve to decrease circulation and warming.

- **Do not overwork the muscles or over-relax the athlete.** Overworked muscles will already be fatigued and not optimized for the event. If the athlete becomes too relaxed, he/she will have a difficult time getting re-energized for the start of competition.

Some athletes prefer not to receive a pre-event massage, since they feel it may interfere with their own preparation routines. Keep in mind that months of preparation can go into an event and that an athlete's final preparation can be ritualistic, eccentric, and even superstitious.

In general, be more conservative with pre-event work so as not to overdo it, especially when working with an athlete for the first time. Avoid any techniques which may require a period of recovery on the part of the muscles (i.e., trigger point work, deep muscle therapy, myofascial lengthening) or anything that may produce pain. This applies to any massage done on the day of the event but can also apply to massage the day prior to the event, or even several days before.

INTER-EVENT MASSAGE

In some sports, athletes will be competing in multiple events within one day. Sports such as swimming and track and field may have individual athletes compete in one event, break for a period of time, and then compete in another event.

Make sure to avoid discomfort and focus on the physical recovery of the muscles used in the previous event. In addition, the therapist must also give attention to the athlete's psychological recovery and help prepare the athlete for the upcoming performance.

Massage applied between events in a single day can have aspects of a post-event massage, a pre-event massage, or both, depending on the timing of the massage in relation to the events.

In general, inter-event massage is brief (10–15 minutes), has the same cautions as a pre-event massage, and is performed during breaks for the athletes. The massage techniques applied depend upon the timing of the massage. The closer an athlete is to the start of an event, the more an inter-event massage resembles a pre-event massage. The further the athlete is from the start of an event, the more the massage resembles post-event treatment.

POST-EVENT MASSAGE

Purpose

The post-event massage is employed after hard training, recreational activity, or competition. It promotes a general state of relaxation, reduces muscle tension, spasm, and cramping, and helps muscles recover more quickly from fatigue. The length of recovery time from strenuous competition can be dramatically reduced with a good post-event massage. Stretching, body mobilization, and techniques that encourage venous and lymphatic circulation are recommended.

In the post-event phase, the muscles are in a state of congestion and fatigue, following maximal performance and exertion. The tissues are saturated with the waste products of intense metabolic activity. Circulatory assistance is needed to speed the elimination of these wastes. Primary techniques are pétrissage, jostling, and compression. The therapist must pay particular attention to the sensitivity and tone of the athlete's muscles, which may vary greatly according to the event and the athlete's condition. Any pressure exerted by the therapist should not cause the athlete pain; pain is definitely unnecessary and counter-productive, adding insult to injury after intense effort by the athlete. Gauge your pressure according to the sensitivity of the muscles, working gradually to loosen and decongest the tissue.

An added purpose of post-event massage is to screen the athlete for injury and potentially dangerous conditions that may result from the competition, assist athlete with specific needs (such as cramping), and make appropriate referrals if necessary. A therapist performing post-event massage must be particularly watchful for signs that an athlete is suffering from conditions that may require specific medical intervention. Therefore, increasing local circulation is an important goal for post-event work.

OVERVIEW

Description—Post-Event Massage Is:

- Non-specific—focus is on major muscle groups used in the event.
- Relatively light—deep techniques are contraindicated.
- Relaxing—focus is on relaxing muscles and athlete as a whole, pace is slower than pre-event.
- Short in duration—10–15 minutes maximum up to one hour after an event.
- Event specific—emphasis is on large muscles used for particular event, especially hypertonic areas
- Painless—no pain should be experienced (deep, digital pressure is contraindicated).
- Pleasing—ideally, the athlete should feel emotionally better after the massage, should be a 'rewarding' experience.

Goals of Post-Event Massage

- Assess athlete's overall condition—using appropriate interviewing and screening techniques to gauge what the athlete's needs are, if he/she need specific assistance, or should be immediately referred for medical intervention.
- Provide general relief from exhaustion.
- Relax tight muscles—help return contracted and/or spastic muscles to normal tone.
- Increase venous and lymphatic circulation and remove post-activity metabolites.
- Relieve muscle cramping if present.
- Reduce post-competition stress. Help create an improved mental state particularly after intense or prolonged activity.
- Provide water or electrolyte replacement if needed.
- Provide appropriate medical referral.

TECHNIQUES

As with pre-event massage, most of the massage techniques you have learned so far can be utilized in a post-event sports massage with the same exception of gliding techniques. However, there are techniques which will be more efficient and effective in the time frame that you have, and certain techniques that you will want to avoid using until you get a sense of how sensitive the athlete's muscles are and whether there is any potential for cramping.

- **Pétrissage**—Your first best bet in post-event work. Pétrissage helps to milk the tissues of metabolites without placing a lot of direct pressure on what might be sensitive muscles.
- **Jostling & Vibration**—Great techniques for inducing systemic or local relaxation when used gently.
- **Compression**—Good for relaxing muscles and promoting circulation, but can only be performed once you have assessed the athlete for soreness and sensitivity.
- **Movement Techniques**—Promotes relaxation and decompression of joints but should only be performed after assessing the tissue for hypertonicity and spasm. Contraindicated if cramping is possible or likely.
- **Gentle Passive Stretches**—Helps return hypertonic muscle to normal length but, like body mobilization techniques (BMT), is contraindicated if cramping is possible or likely.
- **Cramp Relief Techniques**—Indispensable when needed.

Effective massage therapy can be performed without requiring the athlete to remove all clothing. Working through running shorts, T-shirts, or even sweat pants should not present a problem. Do not have the athlete remove his or her shoes.

CAUTIONS

All the normal contraindications are to be respected in a post-event massage. There are also a few specific cautions to be considered:

- **Do not work on a 'hot' athlete.** The athlete must have taken time for an appropriate cool-down prior to receiving massage. Heart rate and blood pressure must be lowered, respiration returned to resting levels, metabolic rates slowed, profuse sweating tapered, and endorphin rush must be diminished. Many post-exercise problems begin to appear during the cool-down and may not have been apparent prior to that, making it difficult to perform adequate screening. An athlete that has over-exerted or needs medical attention may not be able to get up after getting on your massage table. A minimum of 15–20 minutes post event cool-down is mandatory prior to receiving massage.
- **Be careful with pressure.** After an event (especially if prolonged or intense), athletes can be very sensitive. Muscles may be extra-sensitive because overuse can traumatize the tissues, and excessive lactic acid and metabolites can irritate nerve endings.
- **No deep or specific work** (trigger point, transverse/longitudinal friction). Even if the athlete has a specific issue or injury, the post-event massage is not the time to work them out. Endorphins in their system makes it impossible to get an accurate gauge of discomfort for deep work, and it takes a couple of days for the full extent of an injury to be known. Working on it prematurely may cause more damage. Since it is very likely that the athlete has had some microtrauma in his/her tissues, we want to be sure that we don't add to the trauma with excessively deep techniques.
- **Do not apply heat.** Heat has the potential to increase inflammation caused by activity. (Mild heat packs may be appropriate only if the athlete is suffering from hypothermia).
- **Do not work on suspected strain, thermal injury, cuts, blisters, bruises, fractures, etc.** Have the athlete seek appropriate medical care. Watch out for areas with bloody abrasions or opened blisters. These types of injuries are very common in runners and triathletes on the feet, nipples, or other areas where rubbing or chafing has occurred.
- Many athletes will use over-the-counter non-steroidal anti-inflammatory drugs (NSAIDs) such as ibuprofen, aspirin and naprosyn to inhibit the inflammatory response.
- **Contract/Relax for stretching is usually avoided because it may induce cramping.**

ATHLETE SCREENING FOR POST-EVENT MASSAGE

One of the most important functions of providing massage therapy in a post-event environment is to screen athletes for injuries and potentially dangerous conditions. It is best to perform this screening prior to the athlete getting onto your table, chair, etc. A tired athlete will want nothing more than to lie down on your table. But, once there, the athlete is in your care. No one should get on your table until you are comfortable with his/her condition and you ask him/her to do so. An athlete on your table with an injury will be much more difficult to move for medical care. Screening the athlete prior to massage will also make it much less likely that conditions will begin to appear while you are working on him/her.

ATHLETE SCREENING PROCEDURE

It is important for the massage therapist to take charge of the situation. The therapist should be confident, letting the athlete know that he or she is in competent hands. The same procedure should be followed with every athlete.

Conduct a brief interview. This is important for gathering information regarding the athlete's condition. It is not unusual for some athletes to be disoriented or temperamental. Knowing this, the therapist should maintain a comforting, helpful, and professional attitude. Help the athlete feel comfortable by asking questions such as:

- What is your name? (then introduce yourself)
- How are you feeling?
- Where did you place in the race/event? Or, how did you do in the race/event?
- How long has it been since you finished? Have you cooled down yet?
- What areas do you feel need particular attention? Are you feeling any pain?
- Have you had any water yet? How much? Would you like anything to drink?
- Electrolyte replacement (Gatorade, Accelerade, etc.)? How much?
- Have you eaten anything? What and how much?
- Are you feeling hot, warm, or cold?
- Let me know if what I'm doing feels good or hurts . . . especially if it hurts.

Conditions and Injuries to Be Aware Of

While working in the post-event setting, you are likely to encounter some conditions that might require first aid. You should be familiar with the following conditions, as well as how to follow up with first aid, massage therapy, or referral to medical personnel. These objectives can be accomplished efficiently if the practitioner is well-informed and has a concise, effective approach with the post-event athlete.

- Nausea
- Cramps
- Muscle strains
- Sprains
- Dehydration
- Thermal injuries (hyperthermia, hypothermia)
- Blisters
- Cuts, bruises
- Fractures

Athlete Interview Overview

- Ask questions to assess the situation and the athlete's condition.
- Remain in control (don't let the athlete take over).
- No person should get on the table until asked to do so by the therapist.

DELAYED ONSET MUSCLE SORENESS: LACTIC ACID VS. MICROTRAUMA

Delayed onset muscle soreness is the pain in muscles that gradually develops within 1–48 hours after strenuous activity. It is characterized by a feeling of stiffness, achiness, and slowed movement.

A major fallacy perpetuated in sports is that lingering muscle soreness after an activity is the result of residual lactic acid in the tissues. Lactic acid is a normal result of cellular metabolism most often associated with anaerobic respiration. In fact, studies have shown that lactic acid is fairly quickly reconverted into energy by the body and does not linger in the tissues for very long.

The real cause of delayed onset muscle soreness is microtrauma to the tissues. In the process of performing at a strenuous level, the stresses placed on muscle and other tissues actually create a profusion of microscopic tears that are not immediately perceived by the athlete. As the inflammatory process proceeds over a period of a couple days, the symptoms of inflammation begin to become apparent. Severe inflammation can be nearly debilitating and will delay an athlete's return to training.

By promoting circulation, massage therapists can hasten the healing process. Cryotherapy is an effective tool to control inflammation, as well.

THERMAL INJURIES

Screening the Athlete

Sports massage practitioners should become familiar with the signs of hypothermia/hyperthermia and be prepared to refer the athlete to the medical unit if necessary.

In order to avoid escalation of symptoms (preventing mild cases from becoming serious), the massage therapist should routinely ask specific questions of the athlete at the finish line, thoroughly screening him or her for signs of thermal injury. If there are any doubts about mental alertness, the therapist should check in frequently through questioning to monitor the athlete's progress.

HYPOTHERMIA

Description: Hypothermia is defined as a body core temperature significantly below 98.6°F due to the reduction of general metabolism in the body's tissues.

Heat can be rapidly lost from the body when heat loss exceeds production. Amateur or novice athletes may be more prone to hypothermia (e.g., the inexperienced runner may go out too quickly in the early miles of a marathon and must slow the pace later on, causing a loss of core temperature as fatigue and exposure kick in).

Weather conditions also affect the athlete's ability to conserve body heat. Wet, cool, and /or windy conditions, as well as radical changes in the weather during the event, are common contributors to hypothermia.

Possible Contributing Factors

- Hunger
- Fatigue
- Exertion
- Injury
- Amount and condition of clothing
- Lack of fluids
- Prolonged exposure to the elements

Progressive Symptoms

1. Constant shivering (as body attempts to generate heat)
2. Freezing sensation in hands and/or feet
3. Slurring of speech
4. Apathy, listlessness, involuntary muscle movement
5. Euphoria, intoxicated appearance
6. Croaking voice, sleepiness, disorientation, combativeness
7. Generalized rigidity of muscles
8. Unconsciousness, abnormally dilated/pinpointed pupils, very slow pulse and respiration (indications of drastic drop in core temperature)

Care of Hypothermic Athlete (Post-Event)

1. Thoroughly screen the athlete with appropriate post-event questions.
2. If there is any indication of disorientation, ask additional questions (How did you place? Where do you live?, etc.).
3. If athlete is not disoriented but is experiencing chills, fatigue, and cold, assist by:
   a. relocating the athlete to a warm area
   b. helping the athlete change into dry clothing
   c. covering the athlete's head, hands, and feet
   d. covering the athlete's body with blankets or additional insulating cover
   e. briskly rubbing the athlete's body (friction creating heat)
   f. giving the athlete warm fluids
   g. proceeding with treatment once the athlete is sufficiently warmed
4. Medical evaluation is needed promptly whenever serious symptoms are present.

Note: Steam is a fast way to warm the blood, thus raising the core temperature. The athlete may choose to breathe steam to decrease recovery time.

HYPERTHERMIA

Description: Hyperthermia occurs when the rate of heat production in the body exceeds that of heat loss, resulting in an excessively high core body temperature. Hyperthermia becomes a problem most typically in hot, humid weather conditions when the athlete's body cannot dissipate the heat produced by normal biological means.

In humid conditions, a vigorously exercising athlete produces heat from contracting muscles at a rate of 15 to 20 times that of basal metabolism. This is a sufficient level to raise the core body temperature by 1°C every five minutes. Thermal receptors in the hypothalamus sense the increased temperature and respond by initiating the evaporation of sweat, the physiological mechanism through which dissipation of heat occurs.

Evaporation of sweat will, however, be very slow on a hot and humid day because:

- Air temperature exceeds body temperature
- Little additional moisture will be accepted into air which is already highly humidified

The net result is increased heat production and decreased heat dissipation, making the athlete vulnerable to dehydration and a continuum of symptoms, beginning with heat cramps (see Continuum of Heat-Related Thermal Injuries, next page).

DEHYDRATION

Description: Dehydration is excessive loss of water from the body. This impairs the athlete's ability to produce sweat, thereby resulting in thermal injury, cramping, and decreased metabolism. Sweat loss during a long event, combined with inadequate fluid replacement, can result in as much as a 6–10% total body water deficit of body weight.

Signs and Symptoms

1. Multiple muscles cramping/going into spasm
2. White film around mouth/under armpits

CONTINUUM OF HEAT-RELATED THERMAL INJURIES

SYMPTOMS	MASSAGE THERAPY APPROACHES
Level 1—Hyperthermia	
Excessive sweating Shivering/chilling Goose pimples Dry skin Nausea Throbbing pressure in head Unsteadiness Extreme fatigue Muscle cramping	Thorough screening Provide fluids Have athlete lie down (if cooled down from event) Cramp relief sequence Cold compress on forehead General post-event work
Level 2—Heat Exhaustion	
Level 1 symptoms presented as a cluster Level 1 symptoms intensified Increased heart and respiration rates Additional shaking and trembling Eyes unfocused Pale grey skin tone Excessive sweating Some disorientation	SUMMON IMMEDIATE HELP! Use ice/cold packs (forehead, neck, armpits, side of hip) Provide fluids Elevate legs Loosen clothing
Level 3—Heat Stroke	
Sharp upgrade of Level 1 & 2 symptoms Aggressiveness Acute confusion Incoherent speech Increased chills, shivering, goosepimples Unconsciousness Collapse Convulsion Cessation of sweating	IMMEDIATE MEDICAL REFERRAL Medical team will: lie athlete down, loosen clothing, elevate legs, cool entire body, provide advanced life support with intravenous fluids, monitoring of vital signs and transport athlete to hospital

MUSCLE CRAMPS

Definition

A muscle cramp, sometimes referred to as a 'charley horse,' is an intense sustained, involuntary muscle contraction. Technically, a muscle cramp is a type of fasciculation—involuntary contraction or twitching of the muscle fibers. What differentiates a cramp from other types of fasciculation is that the muscle can remain contracted to its full capacity for an extended period with no voluntary control.

As such, a cramp is usually an unpleasant experience. During a cramp, the individual will usually feel it come on suddenly or, in some cases, there may be some anticipatory twitching in the muscle. The muscle itself may feel like it is knotted into a ball, locked in spasm, with no way to stop it. Muscle cramps are usually uncomfortable or even painful, and the cramp may last for a few seconds to a few minutes. In extreme cases, such as cramps resulting from dehydration, episodes of cramping can last for much longer periods of time and might recur multiple times before they cease.

Cramps occur most commonly in the muscles of the lower extremity, thighs, calves, or hamstrings, but can occur in nearly any skeletal muscle. Muscles that span two joints, such as the gastrocnemius, hamstrings, or quadriceps, are the most prone to cramping; however, cramping in the feet, hands, arms, abdomen, and rib cage are also common. Cramps can involve part or all of a muscle, or several muscles in a group.

Signs/Symptoms

The signs and symptoms presented by someone experiencing a cramp are usually fairly obvious.

1. Intense, sudden pain in the muscle

2. Visible and verbal expressions of pain and discomfort

3. Physically holding of the affected area and overall rigidity in the body

4. Decreased movement or joint held in flexion for a prolonged period

5. Local tenderness at the site of the cramp

6. A knotted, hard, balled-up muscle may be visible under the skin

Etiology

The physiology of muscle cramps is not well understood. Because muscle contraction is initiated by motor neurons, a cramp results from abnormalities in the mechanisms that control muscle contraction. Since cramps are involuntary, circumstances in the body are such that there is excess neurological excitation or irritation, enough to alter spinal neural reflex activity and initiate contraction independently. Potential causes of this irritation or excitation are discussed in the next section.

In most cases, a cramp is isolated to muscle bellies or fibers that are connected to one particular motor neuron. However, in cases where the cause of cramping is systemic, the number of motor neurons and muscles involved may be numerous.

Most cramps are painful but not health threatening. Especially forceful or prolonged cramps can result in muscle strain and a need for care, treatment, and rehabilitation. Cramps that are the result of other health issues need to be evaluated and treated by appropriately trained professionals.

CONTRIBUTING FACTORS

The reasons that the neurons initiate and sustain a cramp can be varied and compound. Most common cramps usually occur as a result of a combination of factors.

1. **Overexertion and muscle fatigue**—Overexertion results from calling upon muscles to perform to the point of exhaustion. Energy reserves and oxygen supplies are depleted, leaving the muscle(s) without the resources it needs to function properly. There is also a build up of metabolites in the tissues (waste products resulting from exercise) which can irritate nerve endings. Poor conditioning or training for the tasks calling upon the body (a sporting event, for example) can make the body more susceptible to fatigue. Muscle fatigue can also result from insufficient intake of calories (the energy necessary for proper muscle function).

2. **Inflexibility and hypertonicity**—Muscles that already have too much tone are more susceptible to cramping. Hypertonic muscles, because of their high state of contraction, tend to fatigue more readily. Inflexible muscles, when called upon to stretch beyond their capacity, will contract reflexively and may, in the proper circumstances, initiate a cramp. Inadequate warm-up and/or flexibility training can set up areas of hypertonicity prone to cramps. Structural and functional musculoskeletal imbalances can result in areas of hypertonicity as well.

3. **Dehydration**—Dehydration is the loss or deprivation of water from the body or tissues. Body fluids can be lost through sweating, vomiting or diarrhea (often related to exercising or working in intense heat). Dehydration can also result from inadequate replenishment of body fluids. Metabolism in the body requires proper hydration. These chemical reactions all require water in some way. When fluid levels are depleted, these body functions cannot take place properly. In muscle tissue this can result in cramping.

4. **Electrolyte depletion**—Often occurring in combination with dehydration, electrolyte imbalance refers to an insufficient supply of diluted salts and minerals in the bloodstream. Electrolytes include sodium, potassium, magnesium, phosphorus, and calcium. A lack of these minerals creates an environment in which muscles do not have the chemical components necessary to function properly and may result in a cramp. Other causes of electrolyte depletion may be inadequate nutrition or an excess of fluid in the body. Hyponatremia results from electrolytes being too diluted in the blood stream.

5. **Extremes of heat and cold**—Environmental factors such as heat and cold can play a role in the development of cramps, especially when combined with other factors and physical activity. People exposed to very hot and humid weather or to extremely cold and wet conditions can have their tissues respond in such a way that cramping can develop.

6. **Inactivity**—Inactivity due to injury, disease, or lifestyle can result in insufficient use of muscles to ensure proper functioning and may result in cramping. Also, muscles that are held in a shortened state (attachments are brought closely together for extended periods) may begin to cramp, especially when an attempt is made to lengthen them once again.

LESS COMMON FACTORS CONTRIBUTING TO CRAMPS

Cramps can also be the result of more serious conditions and could relate to problems with circulation, nerves, metabolism, hormones, medications, or nutrition.

- Amyotrophic Lateral Sclerosis (ALS or Lou Gehrig's disease)
- Radiculopathy or spinal stenosis—spinal nerve irritation/compression or narrowing of the spinal canal
- Ateriosclerosis
- Pregnancy
- Thyroid disease
- Chronic infections (such as tetanus)
- Drugs such as lithium
- Cirrhosis of the liver (often a result of chronic alcohol abuse)
- Inflammatory disorders such as polymyositis

See your doctor if cramps are severe, happen frequently, respond poorly to simple treatments, or are not related to obvious causes like strenuous exercise.

Who Is Susceptible To Cramps?

Most people have had a cramp at one time or other. Infants, children, and the aged are more susceptible to heat-related injuries and dehydration. Those suffering from disease, obesity, or who take medications are also at risk. Endurance athletes (marathoners and triathletes) very commonly get cramps due to the nature of their sports and the demands they are placing on their bodies.

Preventing Cramps

Following these guidelines can diminish the possibility of experiencing cramping:

- **Stretching**: a regular program of flexibility exercises can greatly decrease hypertonicity in muscles, provide for better muscle balance, and decrease susceptibility to cramp.

- **Nutrition and Electrolyte Replenishing**: ensure that your body has enough calories for the level of activity it is engaged in and that you have an appropriate intake of essential vitamins and minerals. If engaged in sports, use of sports drinks and carbohydrate replenishment can be very helpful.

- **Hydration**: drinking enough fluids and maintaining proper fluid balance in the body is important for all physiological function.

- **Training and Conditioning**: exercise is important for wellness and health. Training and conditioning is making sure your body is prepared for the stresses that you are going to be placing on it. Conditioning is important for meeting everyday stresses in addition to preparation for a specific sport or activity.

- **Warm-Up and Cool Down**: gradually transition from less activity to greater activity and back again. Engaging in activity too quickly does not allow your body to be properly prepared for the demands placed upon it. Ending activity too quickly diminishes the body's ability to replenish energy stores and remove metabolites from the tissues. It also results in very quick drops in heart rate and blood pressure.

CRAMP RELIEF

It is not uncommon for sports massage therapists to encounter athletes who are experiencing cramping. The high level demands of performance and training, competition, environmental factors, and high metabolism can all combine to make the athlete more susceptible to muscle cramps. Poorly conditioned athletes who compete beyond their level of training can be especially prone to cramps.

Massage therapists might most likely encounter a person with muscle cramps when performing post-event massage. However, any client can develop a cramp during any type of massage. The following cramp relief techniques can be applied to all clients including the athlete.

CRAMP RELIEF TECHNIQUES

There are five primary techniques a massage therapist can employ to assist a client in overcoming a muscle cramp. They are listed here in order of their usual effectiveness from greater to lesser. However, in some cases you may need to employ multiple techniques or circumstances may be such that you may be limited in the techniques you can put to use. In any case, it is important that the massage therapist thinks creatively and acts quickly when a client experiences a cramp.

Intervention Methods for Cramping

1. **Reciprocal inhibition**—The muscle-energy technique reciprocal inhibition may be used to overcome a cramp.

   - **Procedure**—The massage therapist applies resistance to the contraction of the muscle or muscles that are the antagonists to the cramping muscle. The contraction may need to be held for a long enough period for the cramping muscle to begin to let go. This contraction phase is followed by the application of passive stretching to the cramping muscle.

   - **How it Works**—Asking the antagonist to contract sends a message to the brain that in order for this muscle to contract, the cramping muscle must relax (its contraction is inhibited).

   - **Effectiveness**—Can be very effective and works rather quickly in many circumstances.

   - **Cautions**—Can lead to multiple cramps in individuals whose cramps have systemic causes such as dehydration. It is possible for both the agonist and antagonist muscles to cramp simultaneously (very unpleasant).

2. **Muscle Spindle Technique**—This technique uses the action of the proprioceptors in the muscle to overcome the contraction reflex.

   - **Procedure**—The therapist places his/her hands on the musculotendinous attachments on either end of the muscle belly. The therapist then applies pressure in toward the belly of the muscle, effectively shortening the muscle further.

   - **How it Works**—When the pressure is applied to the ends of the muscle belly, shortening the muscle beyond that created by the cramp, it resets the proprioceptors and allows the nervous system to recognize that contraction is no longer needed.

   - **Effectiveness**—Can be very effective, but usually takes a while for the proprioceptors to reset and for the nervous system to respond.

   - **Cautions**—Can be physically demanding to hold the ends in a shortened state for a long period of time. Use good body mechanics and don't overexert yourself. May be slower than reciprocal inhibition.

3. **Direct Sustained Compression**—With this technique, the therapist applies direct compression to the exact site of the cramp for a period of time until the cramp is released. Often, creativity needs to be used to figure out how to apply the compression directly. The client may not be ideally positioned and may be in too much pain to change position. Compression can be applied with palm, fist, knee, thigh, forearm, etc.

   - **How it Works**—Direct compression to the site gives new input (stimulation) to the nervous system, overriding the prevailing contraction reflex.

   - **Effectiveness**—Can be very effective, but usually takes a while for the nervous system to respond. It is great in situations where other techniques are not possible, or if you need to do 'something' while figuring out more advanced techniques to apply.

   - **Cautions**—Compression must be on the exact site of the cramp, otherwise it will not be effective. The cramping muscle may be too painful to apply very much pressure. Exercise care with the amount of compression being applied. In cases of severe cramping where immediate relief is needed, it may be too slow. It can be physically demanding to hold compression for a long period of time. Use good body mechanics and don't overexert yourself.

4. **Ice**—Direct application of an ice pack or ice massage to the cramping muscle can effectively overcome the cramp reflex.

   - **How it Works**—The cold from ice acts as an anesthetic, deactivating the proprioceptors and slowing down the firing of the motor neurons.

   - **Effectiveness**—Can be effective, but it may take a long time for the cold to penetrate deep enough to affect the cramping muscle. Ice may not always be available. The effectiveness of ice can be increased when combined with the simultaneous application of direct sustained compression.

   - **Cautions**—May not be as effective on cramps that are deep in the muscle tissue or on those with a lot of adipose tissue. Do not use with individuals suffering from hypothermia.

5. **Stretch**—Attempt to apply a passive stretch to the cramping muscle.

   - **How it Works**—Basically, attempting to elongate the contracting muscle may be enough to signal the cramp to end, and for the muscle to begin to relax.

   - **Effectiveness**—Not always effective. A cramping muscle may actually elicit more pain if an attempt to stretch it is performed. Can be very effective when the muscle has begun to let go of its own accord or due to some other cramp relief technique.

   - **Cautions**—Too much forceful stretching may cause injury to the muscle.

Note: Unless there is an injury, stretching the muscle after the cramp has abated is useful in preventing a return of the cramp, to help the muscle return to its normal length, and to promote normal function. However, premature stretching can irritate the muscle again, sending it back into cramp. Make sure that the cramping reflex is gone by moving into a stretch very slowly and checking in with the client to see if he/she feels the cramp returning.

Reciprocal Inhibition Procedure for Cramp Relief

Quadricep (Seated)

Client's Position: Seated. Leg is probably straight or slightly flexed at the knee.

Contraction Phase

1. Kneel in a lunge position facing the client.

2. Stabilize behind the client's ankle with both hands. Ask the client to flex the knee joint by pulling his/her heel toward the buttocks as hard as he/she can, thus activating the hamstring muscles.

Note: If the client cannot bend the knee:

- Support the leg under the knee and ankle, and raise the leg slightly upward.

- Ask the client to extend the hip by pulling his/her leg down toward the ground, activating the hamstring muscles.

Stretch Phase

1. Kneel in a lunge position facing the client.

2. Stabilize the straight leg just proximal to the posterior aspect of the knee joint with your superior hand; your inferior hand is on top of the ankle.

3. Flex the knee by sliding or pushing the foot toward the client's hip. At first the stretch may only unlock the knee joint into flexion.

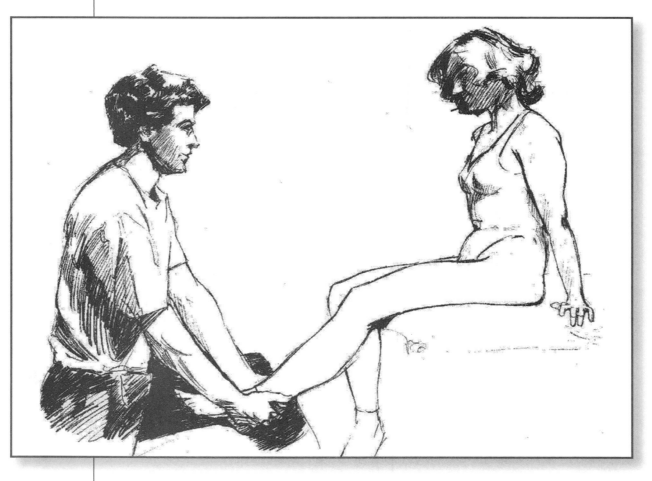

Reciprocal Inhibition Procedure for Cramp Relief

Hamstring (Seated)

Client's Position: Seated. Knee is probably bent.

Contraction Phase

1. Kneel in a lunge position facing the client.

2. Stabilize proximal to the knee joint with one of your hands; the other is placed in front of the ankle. Ask your client to extend the knee joint by pushing his/her foot outward toward your hand, thus activating the quadriceps muscles. Note: During the Contraction Phase you may need to stabilize with both hands in front of the ankle.

Stretch Phase

1. Kneel in a lunge position facing the client.

2. Stabilize the leg just proximal to the posterior aspect of the knee joint with your superior hand and behind the ankle with your inferior hand.

3. Extend the knee by pulling the ankle outward, away from the client.

Considerations

When the client is seated, the client resists by pushing the ankle/foot upward (leg extension). The therapist facilitates the stretch phase by pulling the client's ankle/foot into extension of the knee.

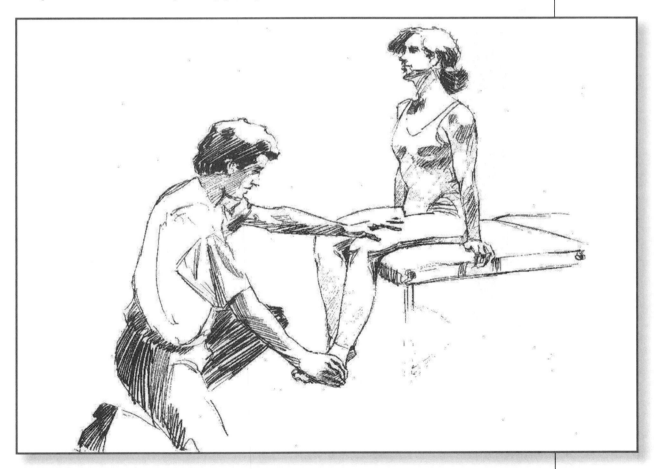

Reciprocal Inhibition Procedure for Cramp Relief

Hamstrings (Prone)

Client's Position: Prone. Knee is bent.

Contraction Phase

1. Stand in a lunge position facing the client.
2. Stabilize proximal to the knee joint with one of your hands; the other is placed in front of the ankle. Ask your client to extend the knee joint by pushing his/her foot toward the table, thus activating the quadriceps muscles. Note: During the Contraction Phase you may need to stabilize with both hands in front of the ankle, as demonstrated in the illustration.

Stretch Phase

1. Stand in a lunge position facing the client.
2. Stabilize the leg just proximal to the posterior aspect of the knee joint with your superior hand and behind the ankle with your inferior hand.
3. Extend the knee by pulling the ankle down toward the table.

Considerations

Make sure not to force this stretch. It may be more effective to ask the client to turn over into supine position for the stretch.

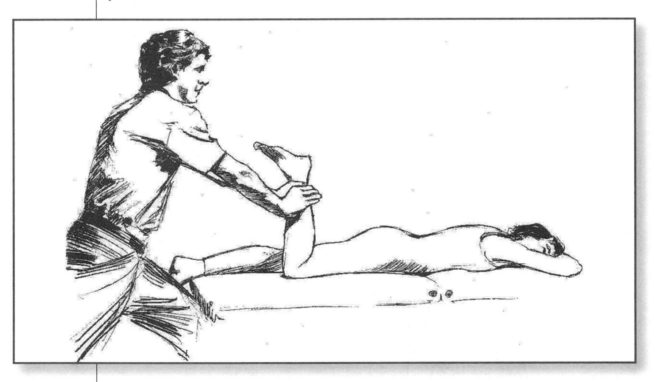

TRAINING MASSAGE

Training massage is an area of specialty unto itself. The approaches that are categorized within training massage can be applied to an individual athlete within a single massage session but are most used in on going sessions.

It is the purpose of this manual to inform the student of the scope and intent of this work. Further training is necessary to adequately meet the needs of athletes on a continual basis. Knowledge of the following will prepare the massage therapist for working with athletes. In effect, these are the preconditions for developing an expertise in the theory and practice of training massage:

1. The physiological effects of sports massage techniques

2. Muscle anatomy, physiology, and kinesiology

3. The normal range of motion of all the major joints of the body

4. The action, origin, and insertion of all the major muscles of the body

5. The pathophysiology of injury and the injury repair process

6. How the massage therapist can positively intervene in the injury repair process

7. Common athletic injuries, including sprains and strains

8. Basic assessment procedures

9. Cryotherapy: the therapeutic use of ice for acute and chronic injuries and for rehabilitation

10. Rehabilitation: massage therapists should be familiar with their unique role in the rehabilitation process and when to refer to other sports specialists

11. Factors that predispose an athlete to injury, such as structural misalignment, overuse, improper or unbalanced exercise, running on hard or uneven surfaces, etc.

12. An understanding of strength training and conditioning principles and their importance in athletic training, rehabilitation, and injury prevention

13. An understanding of the areas of the body that are stressed by a particular sport

14. Injury prevention: the benefits of regular massage maintenance

In the best circumstances, the massage therapist is part of a 'team' or group approach to the athlete's training, including coaches and trainers, rehabilitation specialists, and nutritionists. All these individuals work together to support the athlete by helping him or her reach the highest levels of performance coincident with his/her most important competitions. It is worthwhile for the sports massage therapist to stay current with trends in sports medicine, sports physical therapy, and athletic training, as this information will help the massage therapist to best serve the athletes needs and to interact appropriately with other individuals supporting the athlete. This can be accomplished through study of various health, sports medicine, and athletic training journals, as well as a comprehensive program of continuing education.

TRAINING MASSAGE DEFINITION

Although it is one of the family of approaches called "Sports Massage," training massage is differentiated from pre- and post-event massage by the fact that it does not normally occur in relation to a single event, but represents ongoing work with an athlete. Training massage is the application of ongoing massage therapy to promote the goals and meet the specific needs of the athlete. Generally, training massage occurs any time an athlete receives massage therapy on a day other than that of an event, competition, or workout day (with exceptions—see "Recovery Massage").

TRAINING MASSAGE OVERVIEW

As stated previously, training massage can be divided into three categories based on intent, goals, and application.

RECOVERY MASSAGE

Usually applied 1–3 days after an event or training session (though with certain precautions may take place the day of an event). Recovery massage shares many of the same goals and cautions as post-event massage but is differentiated by the fact that it does not usually take place immediately after an event and may be longer in duration.

Intent

The general intent of recovery massage is to promote the processes that assist the body in returning to normal function and status after strenuous exertion.

Goals

- Increase circulation to promote healing—promotes the healing process by forcing metabolites out of the tissues and increasing the circulation of the resources needed for healing.

- Return muscles to normal tone. Decrease any tendency of the body towards spasm or hypertonicity.

- Decrease delayed onset muscle soreness.

- Decrease any inflammatory processes that may be present. Uncontrolled inflammation will tend to increase recovery time. The application of massage and cryotherapy techniques to control inflammation will facilitate a quicker return to training. This includes decreasing edema and facilitating movement without pain.

- Promote general relaxation. Relaxation is central to any healing process.

Application

The areas of the body most stressed by the activity receive the bulk of the attention. Techniques that increase circulation are of primary importance, i.e., gliding and draining strokes. Mild movement and stretching can be very beneficial as well, to help muscles relax and lengthen. More specialized approaches, such as lymphatic drainage, can be beneficial if edema is present, but require advanced training. Jostling and rocking are good techniques to encourage 'letting go' of tension, and when muscles are held unconsciously. General massage techniques to promote relaxation should be incorporated to enhance the healing process. To enhance the therapeutic effects of this type of massage, the athlete can spend time beforehand in a hot shower, whirlpool, sauna, or steam room.

Contraindications/Cautions

Be cautious with pressure. Muscles may be sore and not tolerant of normal amounts of pressure. Depending on the severity of the need for recovery, care must be taken not to overwork the tissues. They are already suffering from pain and fatigue and there are limits to the amount and degree of massage that can be applied with positive benefit. It is important to be aware that sometimes it takes time for an injury or complication to manifest after the athletic event. Therefore, deep work is usually contraindicated.

Note: It is possible to apply recovery massage the day of an event with particular focus on relaxation and promoting circulation. Special care must be taken in terms of pressure and not doing too much due to the fact that many injury or inflammation processes, if present, will not have had time to develop.

MAINTENANCE MASSAGE

Maintenance massage is the application of ongoing massage therapy to promote the goals and meet the specific needs of an athlete in training. Generally, maintenance massage occurs any time an athlete receives massage therapy on a day other than that of an event, competition or workout day.

Intent

To generally meet the ongoing needs of the athlete with specific attention to the areas most commonly stressed by the sport/training or areas of known difficulty. Techniques are applied that maintain the athlete's body and tissues at an optimal level. It is also possible to do some experimentation with the idea of improving tissues or expanding abilities. This might include breaking up or releasing adhesions and fibrosis, deactivating trigger points, increasing ROM, making postural improvements, releasing hypertonic muscles, etc.

Goals

- To keep the recipient in an optimal condition as he/she is training and to maximize the benefits of rest. Because he/she recover more fully, he/she train more consistently and at higher levels, resulting in enhanced performance on the day of the event.

- Assisting with whatever specific goals have been set by the coach, trainers, etc., such as improved flexibility, kinesthetic awareness, or relaxation.

- Assessing the athlete's body for potentially developing problems or imbalances that may lead to injury. Addressing those problems before they can become a factor in the athlete's training. During a session a therapist is looking for unhealthy tissue—assessing the tissues in areas of high risk for the individual and his/her sport. The primary goal here is to maintain healthy tissue and prevent overuse injuries from occurring. Tenderness in a muscle, tendon or ligament can be warded off and treated before a problem can occur.

Application

Can include or incorporate many types or forms of bodywork. Some especially effective techniques include:

- Compressive effleurage
- Compressive pétrissage
- Transverse & longitudinal friction
- Muscle Stripping
- Trigger point procedures
- Passive stretching
- Active Assisted Stretches (tense/relax & reciprocal inhibition)
- Thermal therapies

Maintenance massage is best applied on an athlete's rest day and is most beneficial if received on a regular basis. A maintenance massage schedule for an athlete is no different than getting your car tuned up on a regular basis. The major impact of the maintenance massage is cumulative changes in the tissue. This is why regular sessions will produce regenerative effects, prevent injuries, and keep the body in optimal condition. The frequency of maintenance massage will depend on the athlete, the sport, the training schedule, and finances.

TREATMENT MASSAGE

Treatment massage is performed when a specific injury is present. It is the specific application of treatment modalities expressly to diminish the effect of the injury and assist in the healing process. These injuries could include strains, sprains, contusions, edema, severe muscle soreness, trigger points, musculoskeletal lesions, adhesions, fibrotic tissue, and chronic inflammatory injuries. Note: just because an athlete has an injury does not mean that he/she may not still be training or participating in his/her sport. Many athletes (especially professional) will continue in the face of injury and wait until the off-season or break to address specific problems. They sometimes will ride a fine line between performing with a condition that is annoying but not completely debilitating, and overdoing it to the point that they are forced by their own body to stop.

Intent

After proper medical attention has been acquired, to facilitate the healing and rehabilitation of injuries through manual intervention.

Goals

- To facilitate the healing and rehabilitation of injuries through manual intervention
- To decrease the inflammatory process
- To intervene in the pain-spasm-pain cycle
- To break up scar tissue and adhesion
- To restore movement, range of motion and function

Application

Treatment massage should usually be applied when someone has an injury but is otherwise not in recovery mode. The therapist and athlete must carefully choose when to pursue rehabilitative measures if the athlete is still training and competing.

Myofascial Massage

INTRODUCTION

Myofascial massage is a manual therapy which can be delivered through a series of designed sessions or as an intuitive selection of techniques, both with an intent to affect the connective tissue of the body. The intent is to realign this connective tissue, freeing it, and thus enhancing its ability to provide structural strength and allow for movement. Fascia, one form of connective tissue, is the enveloping medium that wraps around all structures of the body, giving them support, form and the essential components for repair. Myofascial massage uses specific techniques to release fascial restriction, allowing the tissue to become more pliable.

The major difference between myofascial massage and foundational massage is that, in myofascial massage, the therapist has to be very focused, centered and patient, and must slow down to 'listen' to the tissues. It is vital for the therapist to work from a strong biomechanical base, as this reduces the physical strain on the therapist, and it allows the therapist to attend to the client while remaining attuned to the subtleties of the work.

This type of massage and its application require the therapist to work with fascia in a manner whereby it has to go through a process of physical change (thixotropy) in order for it to elongate, unwind and release adhesions. Certain tissues require a form of external influence to change their molecular composition from a harder solid into a softer substance. The influencing factors can take on many different forms, such as heat from thermal applications, heat from friction, heat from the person's own metabolism, heat applied by mechanical forces through compression and/or stretching, and energy found in energetic bodywork modalities. This process of change described above takes time to happen if it is to be effective in the release of stuck, matted and fibrotic areas.

Myofascial massage requires a change in the therapist's concept of massage application. In typical foundational massage, the engagement tends to be more rhythmical in pressure, lighter at first, then proceeding deeper, back to lighter, and transitioning out. With myofascial techniques the engagement needs to be held steady and on one singular horizontal plane. Along with patience to hold steady engagement, allowing time for the molecular process called thixotropy to take place, during the myofascial technique application it may seem as though nothing is taking place. It might not have the same sense of massage gratification to the receiver as foundational massage.

The intent of these techniques is not to increase circulation, mimic muscle contraction, move venous and lymphatic fluid, or to break up hypertonicity in musculature. Instead, these positive effects are secondary effects due to the release of fascia that can entrap blood vessels, lymphatic vessels, nerve fibers and constrict muscle fibers.

In the typical myofascial massage, the therapist:

- Uses no lubricant for this work
- Does the non-lubricated work first when integrating modalities (the student will practice this in MAS139)
- Identifies what areas need to be worked
- Determines positions the client will assume, in order to most efficiently access those tissues involved (supine, prone, sidelying, seated)
- Chooses what techniques are appropriate for the area to be most effective

HISTORY

The history of myofascial massage goes back to the 1930's. Elizabeth Dicke, a German physiotherapist, developed the Connective Tissue Manipulation technique ('bindegewebsmassage') in 1938. Its focus was working with the superficial fascia, the skin and reflexes to affect other parts of the body.

Ida Rolf was a biochemist who received her Ph.D. from Columbia University and developed Structural Integration during the 1950's–1960's. Her approach focused on the client's proper vertical alignment and releasing the adhesions that constrict and shorten posture. She developed a specific ten-session protocol to work systematically through the entire body. This approach became known as Rolfing©.

John Barnes, a physical therapist, used myofascial techniques during the 1970's and 1980's to relieve pain, restore function and mobility and release emotional trauma. This approach integrated the concept of emotions and memory being stored in the connective tissues (fascia), which contributes to structural dysfunction. He trademarked the term Myofascial Release (MFR)™.

Tom Myers, who was trained by Ida Rolf, has divided the fascial system into ten meridians called Anatomy Trains. He teaches that fascia has specific superficial and deep fascial anatomy meridians that run along the body, and these fascial 'lines' are connected physically and kinesthetically. Dysfunction anywhere along one aspect of the line will have effects throughout the entire line. He uses the concept 'tensegrity', a term coined and developed by Buckminster Fuller, regarding how myofascial techniques work with the structure of the body through this principle of tensegrity.

PRACTICAL APPLICATION

Purpose

The purpose of Myofascial massage is to provide real and long-lasting tissue change for the benefit of a client's well-being. Many of our clients suffer from chronically stressed and painful tissues, and their myriad postural distortions combine to prevent them from enjoying the full use of their bodies. They are the 'vertically ill', moving through life with physical restrictions and limitations, whether from structural origins or postural perpetuating factors. They are the ideal candidates to receive Myofascial massage, as this modality offers the possibility of affecting change in the body by freeing fascial restrictions, elongating shortened muscle fibers, and increasing mobility to inflexible structures.

Myofascial massage uses slow, gentle, mindful and exploratory techniques with subtle and incremental pressure, making it an ideal therapy for clients who are unable or unwilling to undergo more vigorous or dynamic techniques. People recovering from accidents or surgery, seniors and/or those clients who prefer a more intuitive approach can all enjoy myofascial work.

Basic Intent

- Remove fascial restrictions and restore normal muscle length ("form" must be changed to change function)
- Rehydrating fascia
- Restore mobility

FUNCTIONS OF FASCIA

1. Filtration
   - Allows for diffusion of nutrients and waste products
   - Can become repository for metabolites and toxins
2. Immune response
   - Resists the spread of bacteria
   - Contains mast cells, macrophages and other white blood cells
   - Is where inflammatory response occurs
3. Kinesthesia
   - Richly endowed with muscle spindles and golgi tendon organs via muscular fascia layers
   - When armored can prevent body awareness
4. Movement
   - Directs the forces generated by muscle contraction across broad planes
   - Allows for independent movement of muscles/organs
5. Pathways
   - Foundation upon which all vessels and nerves follow
6. Connection
7. Protection
   - Meninges, etc.
8. Repair
   - Most tissue inflammatory response and rehabilitation occurs in the fascia
9. Support
   - Hydrostatic
   - Tensegrity
10. Tonus

INDICATIONS

When is myofascial work indicated?

Complaints of chronic pain, tension or heaviness, loss of range of motion, shortened or warped myofascial structures, distortions in posture or gait, hard, unmoving or traumatized tissue—all of these can be indications for myofascial massage therapy.

This work can create change on a deep, profound level. It can free holding patterns of long-standing duration. It can alleviate pain, even—or especially—that deep ache that is chronically lingering in the background, only to flare up periodically and relentlessly.

Myofascial massage therapy can assist a person into full reintegration of, and with, their body. As restrictions are released, it can help the parts work together as a whole in beautifully balanced, cooperative movements. It can also help with a re-owning of body segments that have been injured, denied, repressed, abused or ignored.

In theory, holding patterns in connective tissue have the potential to store emotional qualities. These emotional qualities may manifest for months or years, and can contribute to tissue restrictions, limiting range of motion, and energy depletion, leading to a pain-spasm-pain cycle (holding pattern-emotional quality-holding pattern). Myofascial work may aid to release these holding patterns.

CONTRAINDICATIONS

Refer to the APP and MAS materials for standard massage contraindications.

- Edema due to acute injury
- Local infection
- Open wounds or fractures
- Degenerative joint disease
    - (Osteoarthritis, chondromalacia, gout, etc.) depends on severity
- Cancer
- Cellulitis
- Aneurysm
- Acute rheumatoid conditions
- Advanced osteoporosis
- Advanced diabetes
- Prolonged use of oral cortisone and cortisone injections

MACRO FASCIAL ANATOMY

Connective Tissue

- Supportive: bone and ligament
- Liquid: blood and lymph
- Connective Tissue Proper: all other connective tissues

Superficial Fascia

Function:

- Provides energy from fat stored
- Provides protection for the skin
- Provides a passage for nerves, blood vessels and lymphatic vessels
- Provides thermal insulation

Deep Fascia

Function:

- Compartmentalizes: cavities, muscle shapes, attachments
- Provides protection for underlying tissues and organs
- Provides a passage for nerves, blood and deeper lymphatic vessels
- Medium for inflammation and tissue repair

Visceral or Subserous Fascia

Function:

- Allows movement of organs
- Allows passage of fluids

Name of Fascial Structures

- Endomysium, perimysium, epimysium
- Tendons, ligaments
- Aponeurosis (tendon in the form of a sheet)
- Retinaculum (thickened component that allows for independent tendon movement)
- Periosteum (layer around bone that serves as attachment for muscles)
- Meninges (layer around spinal cord and brain)
- Meniscus (supports and protects joints)
- Joint capsule (encloses joints and houses synovial membranes for free joint movement)
- Bursae (houses synovial membranes for tendon protection)

RELEVANT FASCIAL STRUCTURES

Dura Mater

Flexor and Extensor Retinaculum

Palmar Aponeurosis

Temporal Fascia—Superficial and Deep

Occipital Frontal Aponeurosis

Ligamentum Nuchae (nuchal ligament)

Pectoral Fascia

Thoracolumbar Aponeurosis

Linea Alba

Rectus Sheath—Anterior and Posterior

Abdominal Wall—Three Aponeuroses
- External Oblique
- Internal Oblique
- Transverse Abdominis

Inguinal Ligament

Sacrotuberous Ligament

Gluteal Aponeurosis

Fascia Latae

Iliotibial Tract

Pes Anserine

Lower Leg Fascial Septums

Peroneal Retinaculum at Ankle

Flexor Retinaculum at Ankle

Extensor Retinaculum at Ankle

Plantar Fascia

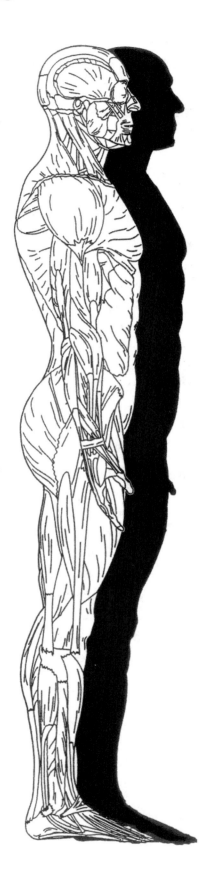

CELLULAR FASCIAL ANATOMY

Fascia Components

1. **Cells:**
   a. Macrophages
   b. Plasma Cells
   c. Mast Cells
   d. Fibroblasts
   - Are the only cells that exhibit a lifelong ability to migrate to any point in the body, then to secrete the specific form of connective tissue needed for repair in that area.
   - Are the earliest specialized cells to emerge from the embryonic mesoderm (human formation)
   - Are able to change their internal structure in accordance to the stress and needs of a particular area-tissue type.
   - Secrete the fluid ground substance and collagen fibers.

2. **Fibers:**
   a. Elastin: Allows for flexibility, can recoil to its rest position
   b. Collagen:
   - Accounts for more then 1/3 of all animal protein.
   - Chief fibrous content of skin, ligament, tendon, cartilage, bone, vessels, and all organs.
   - Strands give to these tissues their shape, tensile strength, resiliency, and structural integrity.
   - Fibers are arranged in numerous ways to produce a wide variety of properties:
     - Criss-crossed randomly in blocks or sheets
     - Stacked in alternating layers like plywood
     - Spun into loose areolar webs
     - Packed into dense parallel forms
   - Tensile pulls determine the amount of strands that twist together and the directional lines into which the collagen fibers arrange themselves.

3. **Ground Substance:**
   - Surrounds all cells in the body.
   - Consistency of the fluid varies from location to location.
   - Allows the passage of gases, nutrients, wastes, hormones, antibodies, white blood cells between the capillaries and the tissues they irrigate.
   - Is both a facilitator and barrier between blood and all the cellular surfaces.
   - Can vary from watery to gel states.
   - Collagen fiber, in various arrangements or amounts, contributes to the make-up the numerous types of connective tissue.
     - watery; little fibers—subserous fascia around organs
     - flexible lattice; less fluid more fibers—fascia around muscles
     - tough stringy material; little fluid many fibers—tendons, ligaments
     - cartilage develops due to chondroblast secretions
     - bone originates as cartilage, which is replaced with mineral salt

Important To Know

Ground substance does not come from capillaries, but is produced by fibroblasts.

Healthy ground substance works constantly to maintain a supportive chemical and physical equilibrium between all the body tissues.

TERMINOLOGY OF FASCIA

Tensegrity Concepts

- Maintain structural integrity by continuously adjusting tension and compression.

- Use poles (bones) and guy-wires (muscle/fascia)

- Tensional force, not compressional strength, keeps a structure rigid

- The tensegrity principle relies on the strength of connecting cables, not the strength of beams

- Bones act more like "spacers" than as compressional members; more weight is actually borne by the connective system of cables than by the bony beams

- Bone would slide off its joint if it were not for the tensional balances that hold it in place

- Buckminister Fuller coined the term 'tensegrity' (maximum stability with a minimum of materials)

- Maladjustments, weaknesses, and imbalances in the lengths and tensions of the cables lead to the instability of the structure (skeleton)

Gel & Sol—state

Gel is when the ground substance is thicker "gelatinous", and sol means more "watery."

Thixotropy

"Turning by touch"—the quality by which fascia goes from gel to sol and sol to gel.

Thixotropy requires energy:

- Heat: sunlight, heat lamps, hydrocollators, baths

- Mechanical (Piezoelectric Concept): quality of change when mechanically compressed, squeezed, stretched

When mechanical stressors are put upon the fascia, it becomes more fluid. When sedate, it becomes more solid.

Example: Right now, students, you are more sedate sitting and listening to this lecture; your fascial structures are naturally becoming more gel-like. When you get up at break and walk around, heat and mechanical pressure are produced, and your fascia will shortly become more sol-like (fluid). Do you notice the change between being a little 'stiff' and losing that 'stiff' feeling shortly after walking around?

Example: Consider gelatin. When it's in the refrigerator, it gels and holds the shape of its container. If it is removed and left to sit in the sunlight, it will slowly melt. Then, if you put it back into the refrigerator, it gels again.

Hydrostatic Pressure

Lacing and squeezing of tough cords around a fluid filled container that turns the container into a cylinder that becomes rigid.

It is important to know that the Abdominal Aponeurosis, along with the Thoracolumbar Aponeurosis and Rectus Sheath, form a fascial 'girdle' for a 'hydraulic lift'.

- Thoracolumbar Fascia and how the erector spinae are encased in them. They themselves function on the principle of hydrostatic pressure
- Transverse Abdominis and Internal Obliques as attaching directly to the Thoracolumbar Fascia.
- External and Internal Obliques with Transverse Abdominis as "becoming" the Rectus Sheath around the Rectus Abdominis
- This layer crisscrosses to be the Linea Alba

Student Exercise: Place soft, light bag of sugar, flour, or bean bag on the top of your head. Walk around the house doing normal activities for a short period of time while balancing the bag on your head. The act of balancing of the bag will tighten the fascial girdle, providing more stability and tone to the core. This exercise was made famous in the movie "My Fair Lady."

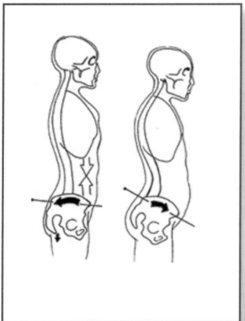
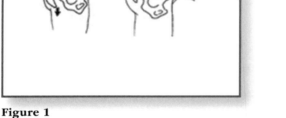

Figure 1

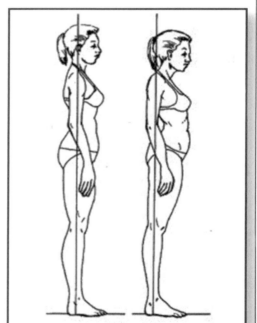

Figure 2

FASCIAL ANATOMY AND PATHOPHYSIOLOGY

Fascial Dysfunction

- Cross-linked fibers (collagen bonding)
- Ground substance thickening (thixotropic properties)

Fascia Encroachment and Constriction

- Nerves, blood vessels, lymphatic vessels
- Ground substance, dehydration

Constriction and Effects of Muscle Tissue Function Factors Affecting Tissue Growth and Plasticity

- Nutrition
- Hormone balance
- Level of physical activity

Fascia in Response To Growth and Stress

Excessive mechanical stress (posture or poor mechanics) can cause excessive deposits of collagen. Thus, restrictions in fascia can lead to limited mobility, postural distortions, poor cellular nutrition, pain, and a variety of other dysfunctions.

Mechanical Stresses

1. Structural Inadequacies
   - Include bony asymmetries that shorten muscles (for example, leg length inequality can cause the pelvis to tilt).
2. Postural Stresses
   - Poor posture: resulting from improperly positioned furniture
   - Poor body mechanics: such as bending/lifting improperly
   - Sustained isometric contraction: such as working at a keyboard for long periods of time
   - Muscle immobility: such as sleeping in a muscle-shortened position, or guarding against pain
   - Repetitive movements: such as playing an instrument or assembly-type jobs (for example, creating coffee drinks)
3. Muscle Constriction
   - Straps of backpack or purse compressing the shoulder or neck

Fascia in Response To Injury

There are two basic types of adhesions

- Layers glued together, much like wrapping tape;
- Layers stitched together: the collagen fibers are the threads (scar tissue)

Fascia and Aging

- Fascia will dehydrate, thicken and crystallize, encroaching on lymphatic, blood, and nerve vessels as we become more sedate
- Elastin loses its quality and becomes "pinned", therefore we lose mobility
- Ground substance loses its thixotropic quality

Basics of Postural Distortions

- In concentrically-held positions, the fascia tends to become glue-like.
- In eccentrically-held positions the muscles can not hold form, therefore the body tends to lay down collagen where it normally does not occur. (This is a simple definition of Fibrosis or Fibrotic Tissue)

POSTURE AND BODY ALIGNMENT

Structural Considerations

The basic structure that support via framework an upright posture in humans is the skeletal system. This system utilizes bones, ligaments, and the gastrocnemius/soleus muscle through the Achilles tendon to direct the forces of gravity along a vertical plane. The natural curves of the spine—cervical, thoracic, and lumbar—allow a hold of the upper portion of the body on a balanced transverse plane, centered at the pelvis.

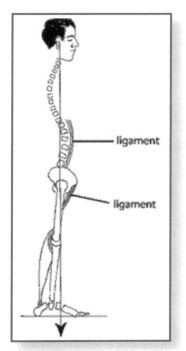

Figure 3a

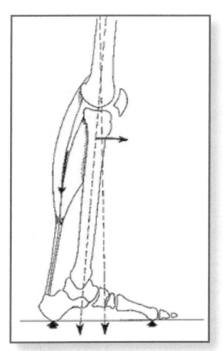

Figure 3b

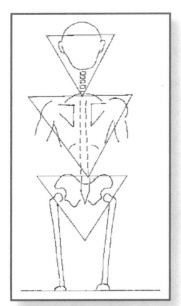

Figure 4

The structure of animals that walk on four legs resembles a simple arch or suspension bridge, designed to bear weight and provide shock absorption for vital organs.

Humans have a bipedal structure that allows optimal freedom of movement for the upper extremities, creating a system dependent upon soft tissue (ligaments, muscles, and fascia) for both support and mobility (tensegrity and hydrostatic pressure).

The human body is divided into three highly movable regions: the head, the torso and the pelvis. The picture of three balanced triangles on their tips illustrates the independent mobility of each region. If humans were designed with an emphasis on stability rather than flexibility and mobility, these three triangles would be reversed, with their bases on the bottom much like a pyramid.

Fascial Considerations

Fascia plays an important role in supporting the musculoskeletal system.

During static upright alignment, the pelvis is balanced horizontally. The tip of the coccyx is level with the top of the pubic symphysis. The weight of the vertebral column and thorax is held plumb over the pelvis by a combination of skeletal curvature, ligaments (such as the iliolumbar ligament), and fascial layers that support the abdominal cavity.

Postural muscles are constantly contracting, subtly, in an effort to maintain balance. For example, the erector spinae group and psoas hold the thorax in the coronal plane, the quadratus lumborum holds the thorax in the sagittal plane, while other muscles contribute to pelvic stability. What supports the muscle tonus, allowing the bones of the vertebral column to carry the weight in gravitational alignment?

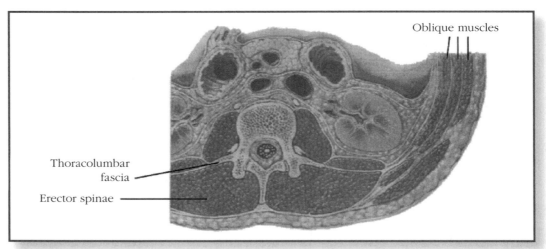

Figure 5
Lumbar Region of the Back (cross section)
©1995 Ciba-Geigy Corp.

The role fascial anatomy plays in the support and alignment of the lumbar region is an essential one. The erector spinae muscles are enveloped in the thoracolumbar fascia. The aponeurosis of the transverse and internal oblique muscles attach directly to the thoracolumbar fascia. The three layers of abdominal aponeurosis continue lateral to anterior, joining together to form the rectus sheath. The rectus sheath envelops the rectus abdominis muscle and joins anteriorly to become the linea alba.

Properly toned muscle and fascia form an envelope around the entire lumber and lower thoracic region creating a hydraulic lift that helps maintain alignment and supports the weight of the upper thorax, shoulder girdle, and head.

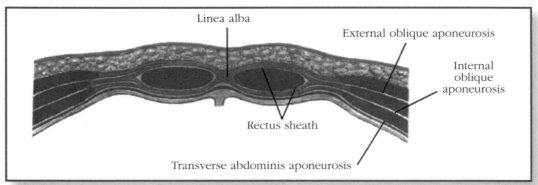

Figure 6
Lumbar Region of the Back (cross section)
©1995 Ciba-Geigy Corp.

MYOFASCIAL MASSAGE THERAPY GUIDELINES

Touching, Connecting, Palpating

- Make gentle contact—resting hands on the body, gentle rocking or compression.

- Enter slowly, until you make contact with a point or areas of resistance (this is the beginning of melting into the tissues).

- Wait.

- Melt (be patient).

- Shift tissues horizontally (take the release horizontally as far as seems appropriate).

- Exit with as much care and awareness as you used when entering the tissues.

Your intent is very important. What does this muscle need? To be softened, lengthened, shifted, unstuck, etc.? What is your postural, motional, and emotional intent?

Generally enter on the client's exhale. Encourage—don't fight—breathing unless you want to stimulate the person.

Don't do anything without feeling what's going on in the body; in deep work, exploration and treatment intermingle. Monitor the person's overall reaction to your work.

Use whole body leverage, not muscular force, for pressure. Grounding your feet, making contact with the floor, is as important as anything your hands are doing.

Pressure should be used to get you to the layer you need to address. Once you reach that level, direction is most important.

Have the client breathe deeply into areas of engagement. Always work cooperatively in regard to pressure, location and duration.

What Are Releases? How Can You Recognize Them?

- A feeling of spaciousness

- A feeling of widening or lengthening

- A settled and relaxed sense of equilibrium

- Respiratory enhancement, change, improvement or deepening

- A sense of unbinding or letting go

- A feeling of pulsation, streaming, or heat

- An existential shift of attitude

DEVELOPING MYOFASCIAL TOUCHING SKILLS

Create an environment of trust and comfort. Place the client in control of the pressure.

Work only with informed consent on vulnerable parts of the body. Stay focused on your intent, and listen to the tissues for feedback. Exit with as much care and reverence as you enter tissue for a maximum effect.

Some Suggestions

- Work superficial to deep. Take your time. Explore mindfully.
- Utilize general contact and warming before proceeding to deeper layers.
- Encourage subtle movements and appropriate breathwork from the client.
- Breathe into tension blocks. Work cooperatively.
- Monitor your angle of entry, and make any directional changes slowly and gently.
- Monitor your biomechanics your own breathing patterns throughout the session.
- After specific areas of body focus, strive for somatic integration—utilizing breath, visualization, or light compression.
- Use a soft hand—probe gently using your hand as a sensor.
- Develop the use of knuckles, forearms, and elbows to intuitively 'feel' tissue changes.
- Working without oil and over clothing may be an ideal option, because you avoid sliding strokes, and must now focus on elements of depth, tissue texture, and areas of tissue alteration.

MYOFASCIAL BODY MECHANICS

Essential body mechanics include a sense of grounding through the legs and pelvis; hips and torso in line with, and facing, your work whenever possible and appropriate; a relaxed and open abdomen, chest and shoulders; and well-aligned wrists and fingers. It is important to assume a comfortable position that will allow for the efficient transfer of body weight into the tissues. Tension or pushing will be easily perceived by the client, and can hinder relaxation and release. Check yourself often for tension, relaxing your neck and shoulders, and repositioning yourself if you become uncomfortable, or if the angle of release in the tissue shifts. Ideal tissue communication is therefore based on ease, intuition, and non-verbal communication.

Pattern of Strain

Techniques delivered with force and effort:

- Fragmented and stressful movements; fighting against gravity
- Body stressfully reacts to hand techniques
- No pain/no gain = ongoing strain
- Attempt to relieve client discomfort by increasing personal effort
- Working with intense focus on body areas that need treatment
- Using force to overcome resistance

Pattern of Ease

Techniques convey a sense of openness and ease:

- Emphasis on pelvis, legs, and feet
- Body moves integratively by working with gravity
- Body initiates actions of the hands and arms
- Ease of therapist results in increase of client's somatic awareness
- Openness to suggestion, relaxation, expanded energetic potential
- Focus on whole body patterns and interweaving
- Respecting body patterns and exploring new options

COMMUNICATION DURING MYOFASCIAL MASSAGE THERAPY

The therapist and client are engaging in a different type of therapeutic relationship in myofascial work. Their intentions and goals need to be shared, and a cooperative method of work is essential. From the beginning, this includes an agreement as to the purpose of the work, the desired outcomes and possible reactions, and a commitment to a general time frame (i.e., five sessions as a start). An ongoing concurrence about physical boundaries is necessary, including areas to be worked or not worked, and bodywork positions considered comfortable.

The therapist needs to formulate a strategic plan to accomplish the desired results, and this is developed from visual, auditory, and palpatory input. While discussing the client's physical history and complaints, many clues will present themselves to an alert therapist: perhaps the sense of energy (or lack of it) overall or in a particular area of the client's body, voice, eyes, etc.; perhaps the client's body language or certain positions of guarding assumed; the tone of voice used, or perhaps even references alluded to. This subtle awareness needs to continue during any body reading or movement assessment that follows, not just noting gross or specific asymmetries, but also an overall view of the person, their energetic levels, and indeed how they might view themselves and relate to the body-mind connection.

The client is an active participant in the therapy and this participation greatly enhances both the physical results of the work and the client's sense of empowerment with their own body, health, and well-being.

Breath and movement are important aspects of the client's role during myofascial bodywork. By encouraging a client to breathe into a site being touched, that will help the softening and release of tissues as the client allows themselves to surrender to sensations.

Breathing also furthers their awareness of the three-dimensionality of the region and its connection to other parts of their physical structure. This in turn helps the person re-energize, re-own, and re-integrate the body part.

TECHNIQUE—HOW YOU DO IT

The diagrams below represent two differing approaches. The dashed line represents the surface of the skin (the dashed line going in a straight line across the page). The solid line shows the pressure and direction of your stroke (the solid line in a wave pattern across the page).

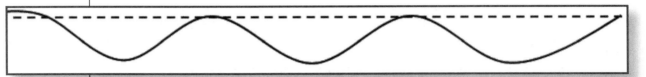

In foundational massage, many of the strokes (particularly the pétrissage category) derive their effectiveness from increasing and decreasing pressure on tissues; or, in the case of friction, by moving back and forth across tissues to produce heat. The strokes can be performed from a slow to a faster tempo and from a light to a deeper pressure. This is the most recognizable form of massage and is used to increase venous blood circulation, help move metabolic waste out of tissues and into the blood stream, decrease hypertonicity, increase relaxation and, when properly applied, help the body to deal with specific conditions.

In fascial release, the goal is to engage the tissue, whether superficial or deep, and affect it with sustained pressure (typically long and slow), providing a plastic change. This sustained pressure needs to follow horizontal lines of engagement thru out the stroke, as oppose to foundational massage as described above, moving in and out, up and down. It requires a different paradigm of thought and intention by the therapist than that of Foundation Massage, that is, the stroke when applied must be set and held at a steady line of engagement. Example is peeling individual layers of an onion.

Fascial release strokes target the connective tissue with the goal of resolving long-term holding patterns, increasing functional range of motion, moving metabolic waste and interstitial lymph through the body and reducing scar tissue or adhesions between layers of connective tissue.

A major course objective is to introduce the student to the different paradigm of technique application, and be patient, not busy.

MYOFASCIAL TECHNIQUE CATEGORIES

General Broad Plane

- Linear Palmar
  - Back
  - Thigh
  - Lower leg
  - Brachial region
- Spiraling
  - Torso
  - Thigh
  - Arm
- Compressive Traction ('S' stroke using palms)

General Deep Plane

- Traction
  - Arm
  - Leg supine and prone
  - Back prone
- Pin and Lengthen
  - Hamstrings
  - Biceps brachii
  - Pectoralis major
  - Quadriceps
  - Neck & upper shoulder

Site Specific

- Skin-Rolling/Shift
  - Back
  - Shoulders
  - Forearms
  - Calves
  - Thigh
  - ('C' and 'S' strokes are variations of this technique)
- Muscle Rolling
  - Trapezius
  - Extensors
  - Deltoids
  - Triceps brachii
  - Latissimus dorsi
- Deep Forearm Gliding
  - Forearm transverse to the region and parallel to the region
- Pin and Mobilization
  - Tendons of greater trochanter
  - Achilles tendon
  - ASIS region in supine
  - Lower leg/ankle retinaculum
  - Wrist retinaculum

Linear Palmar Technique on the Back

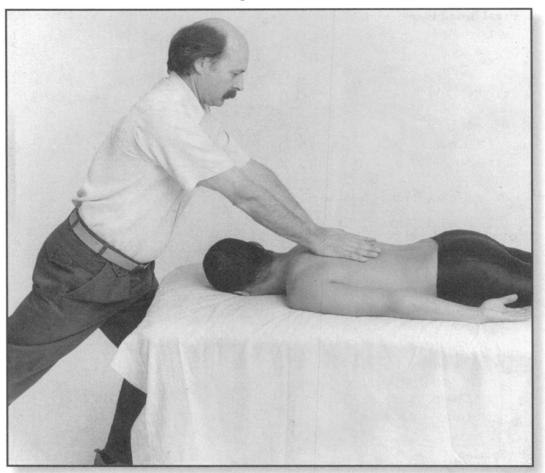

Performance Highlights

- The therapist stands in a low lunge position facing the client's feet. Using a broad surface contact on your palm and fingers, shift the skin to the resistance barrier.

- Holding the resistance barrier, shift your body weight to change the tempo, direction, and to encourage the resistive areas to heat up and release.

- While maintaining your contact, slowly raise and lower your lunge position to change the technique, differentiating from myofascial and slow gliding techniques.

- Also, ask the client to take in a deep slow breath while holding the engagement; then, upon the slow exhale, note the fascial release that may take place.

Spiraling Technique on the Torso

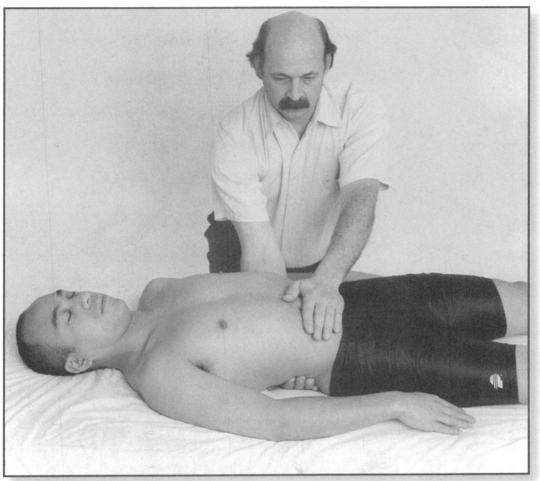

Performance Highlights

- The therapist stands in a low lunge position, or kneeling at the side of the table, facing the lateral border of rectus abdominis. Place your inferior hand on the top and your superior hand underneath the back.

- Using the transfer of your body weight, pull with the hand under the back while simultaneously pushing, or rolling, the hand that's on the abdomen.

- This will be like spinning a large cylinder or drum.

- Sometimes, the lighter the hold, the better the technique.

- While maintaining engagement, ask the client to do a slow pelvic tilt. This will increase the engagement and help to release the tissue.

- CAUTION: this is a horizontal type movement, avoid digging or inward pressure into the torso.

Spiraling Technique on the Thigh

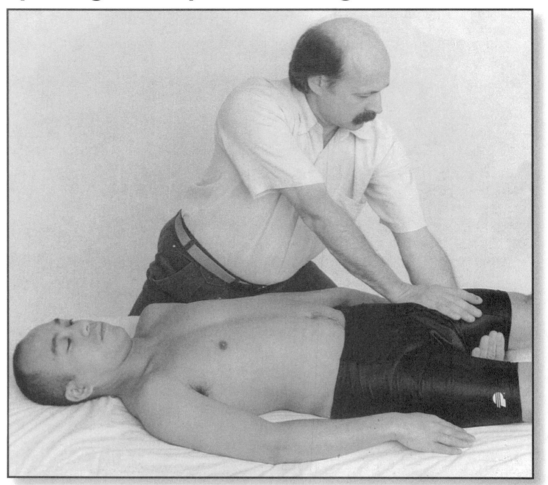

Performance Highlights

■ The therapist stands in a low lunge position, or kneels at the side of the table, facing the client's feet. Place your inside hand on the top of the thigh and your outside hand underneath the thigh.

■ Using the transfer of your body weight, pull with the hand under the thigh while simultaneously pushing, or rolling, the hand that's on top.

■ This will be like spinning a large cylinder or drum.

■ Sometimes, the lighter the hold, the better the technique.

■ While maintaining engagement, ask the client to do a slow pelvic tilt. This will increase the engagement and help to release the tissue.

Spiraling Technique on the Arm

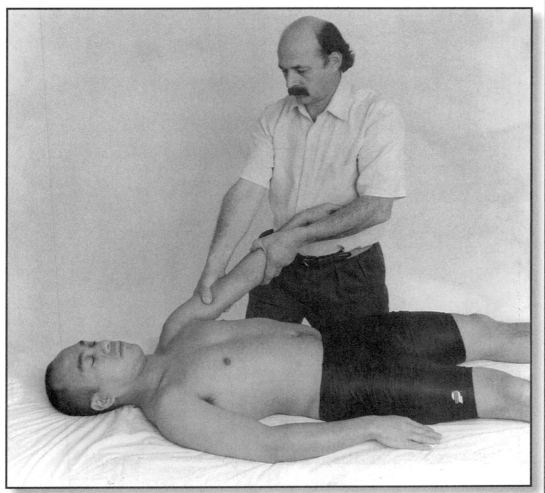

Performance Highlights

- The therapist stands in a lunge position. Place your inside hand around the client's forearm, and your outside hand around the upper arm near the deltoid tuberosity.

- Slightly twist the entire arm, your hands moving in opposite directions (this is not a "burning the skin" technique).

- Use the transfer of your body weight by imagining yourself falling backward, allowing the arm to slightly traction.

- The lighter your hold, the better the technique.

- At first, the feeling is that nothing is happening. Give it time. Imagine you are slowly pulling off a woman's long silk glove.

Compressive Traction on the Back Unilaterally

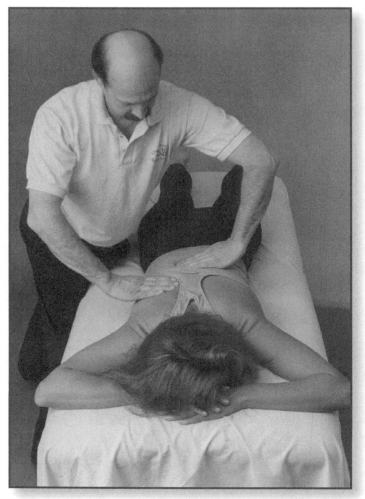

Performance Highlights

- The therapist faces toward either the client's head or feet; shift your body position to be over the client's back on the side you are standing.

- Your fingers, or your palm, should be parallel to each other on the side you are standing, with enough distance between them to allow the tissue to lift without pinching the skin.

- Using a horizontal shifting of the skin, lift the skin in an 'S' shape manner.

- NOTE: this technique is over the erector spinae, not the lateral ribs.

Compressive Traction on the Back Bilaterally

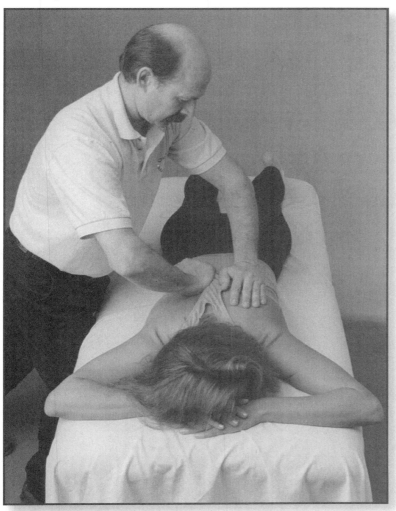

Performance Highlights

- The therapist stands in a low lunge position facing laterally into the client's body. Place your fingers, or palms, on both sides of the spinous processes.

- Your fingers, or your palm, should be parallel to each other with enough distance between them to allow the tissue to lift without pinching the skin.

- Using a horizontal shifting of the skin, lift the skin in an "S" shape manner.

- By switching the hands, the 'S' shape will switch directions.

- NOTE: this technique is over the erector spinae, not the lateral ribs, and the therapist is not thrusting, but horizontally sliding the tissue in both directions.

Compressive Traction on the Thigh

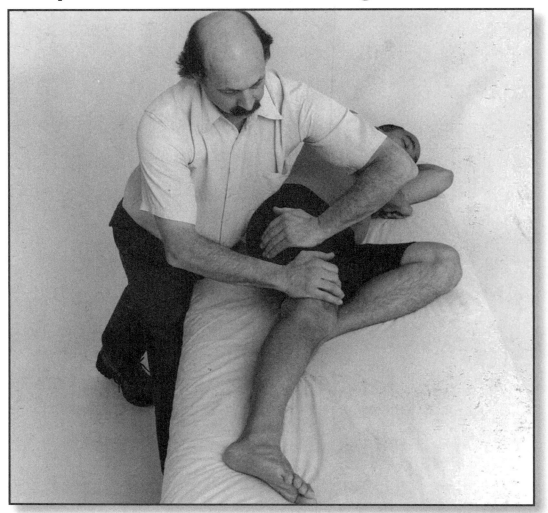

Performance Highlights

- The therapist faces toward either the client's head or feet, shift your body position to be over the client's thigh on the side you are standing.

- Your fingers, or your palm, should be parallel to each other on the side you are standing, with enough distance between them to allow the tissue to lift without pinching the skin.

- Using a horizontal shifting of the skin, lift the skin in an 'S' shape manner.

- NOTE: this technique is over the vastus lateralis, lifting the iliotibial tract off the underlying musculature. Also, switching hands will switch the direction of the 'S' lift.

Pin and Lengthen the Hamstrings

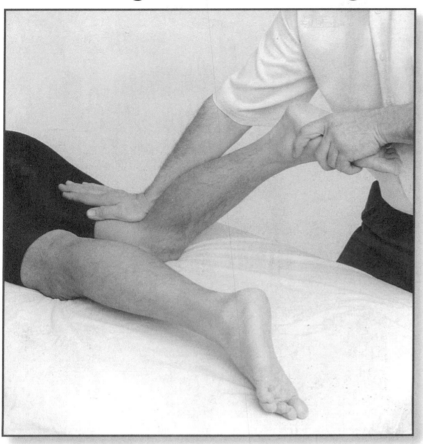

Performance Highlights

- The therapist stands in a low lunge position facing the client's hip. Pick up the client's foot with your inferior hand, flexing the client's knee. Place your palm just proximal to the back of the knee, facing the fingers toward the client's ischial tuberosity.

- Apply a slow upward pressure while simultaneously lowering the foot toward the table. This will create a lengthening effect to the hamstrings.

- Each hamstring can be isolated individually.

- CAUTION: your pressure should not be downward into the leg, but horizontal to the region. Be sure to shift the tissue horizontally until reaching the stretch barrier, then hold that barrier while performing the technique.

Pin and Lengthen the Biceps Brachii

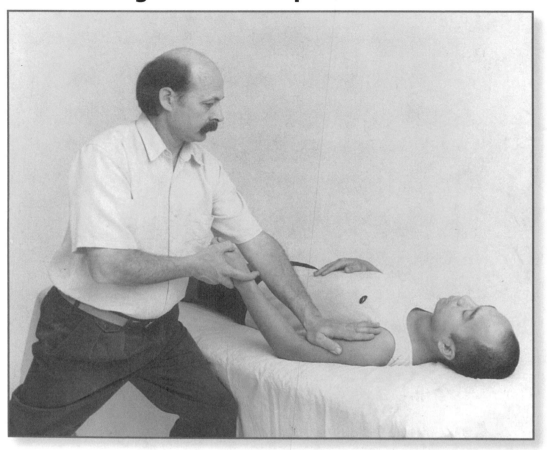

Performance Highlights

- The therapist faces toward the client's shoulder, holding the client's hand in one hand while applying a palmar lengthening to the biceps brachii muscle with the other. Be sure the client's humerus is not medially rotated on the table, that the muscle is straight up toward the ceiling.

- Using your lunge position and simultaneously lowering the client's forearm to the table, slowly glide along the musculature.

- You may choose to use your thumb, applying slow deep thumb lengthening.

- CAUTION: this technique should not produce nerve like referral pain. Be careful of the direct pressure downward into the table.

Pin and Lengthen the Pectoralis Major or Minor

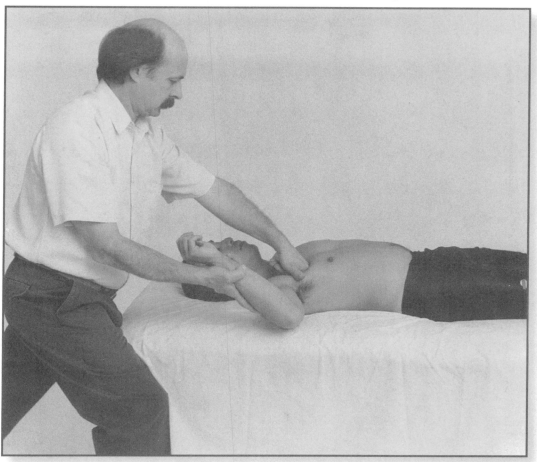

Performance Highlights

■ The therapist stands in a low lunge position at the head of the table. Place a loosely held fist just below the coracoid process of the scapula (attachment site for pectoralis minor). You may choose to use fingertips. Use the transfer of your body weight in an inferior direction; stay soft in your knees.

■ Your inside hand should be stationary during the technique. Your outside hand holds the client's wrist or forearm, while slowly gliding the client's arm in an upward direction. NOTE: keep the client's humerus on the table, allowing it to glide.

■ This technique pins the pectoralis minor as it is elongating into a stretch.

■ CAUTION: if the client feels pain go slower, or change your engagement to a different contact surface.

Skin Shifting and Rolling the Back

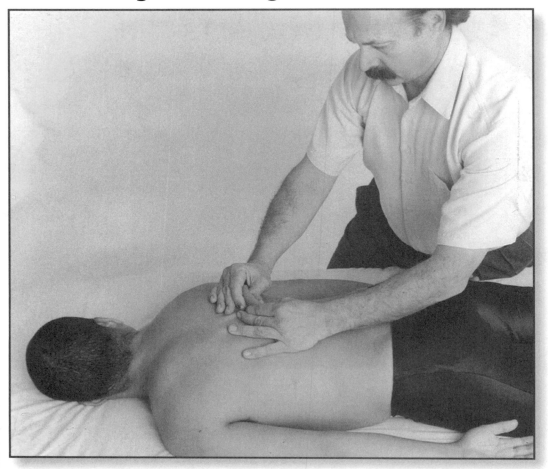

Performance Highlights

- The therapist stands in a low lunge position. Lift the client's skin by gathering it up until you feel the resistance barrier.

- Your hands should be open, with the outside of your palms touching the client. Your contact should always be at the 'base of the wave.' As the tissue releases, it will allow for more skin to be lifted. Be sure to periodically re-gather the tissue.

- Prior to rolling the tissue between your fingers and thumb, shift along the underlying musculature by transferring your body weight to pull in different directions.

- CAUTION: if the client feels pain, go slower, or just use sustained holding with no movement. This will be just as effective for a fascial release.

Skin Shifting and Rolling the Obliques

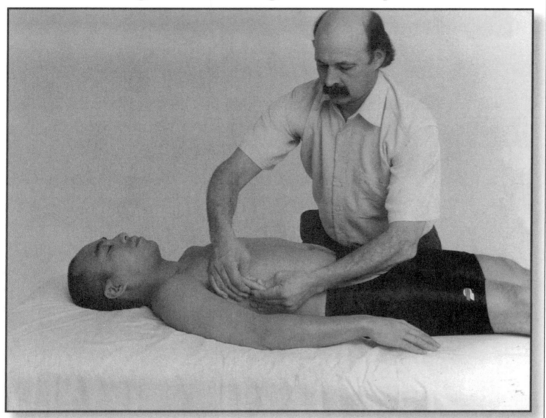

Performance Highlights

- The therapist stands on the opposite side in a lunge position. Lift the client's skin by gathering it up until you feel the resistance barrier.

- Your hands should be open, with the outside of your palms touching the client. Your contact should always be at the 'base of the wave.' As the tissue releases, it will allow for more skin to be lifted. Be sure to periodically re-gather the tissue.

- Prior to rolling the tissue between your fingers and thumb, shift along the underlying musculature by transferring your body weight to pull in different directions.

- CAUTION: if the client feels pain, go slower, or use just sustained holding with no movement. This will be just as effective for a fascial release.

C Stroke Technique on the Lateral Thigh

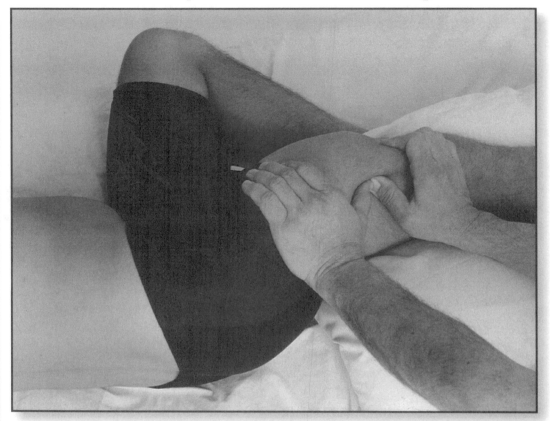

Performance Highlights

- The therapist stands in a low lunge, or kneeling position. Place your fingers posteriorly to the iliotibial tract, with your thumbs under the band. Slowly lift the band off the vastus lateralis muscle by using your arms for leverage, much like doing the 'chicken dance.'

- This technique is similar to breaking a twig or branch of a tree.

S Stroke Technique on the Thigh

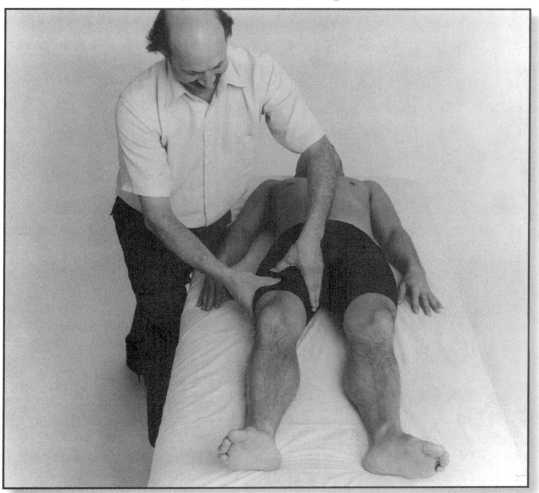

Performance Highlights

- The therapist faces toward either the client's head or feet. Shift your body position to be over the client's thigh on the side you are standing.

- Your fingers, or your thumb, should be parallel each other on the side you are standing, with enough distance between them to allow the tissue to lift without pinching the skin.

- Using a horizontal shifting of the skin, lift the skin in an 'S' shape manner.

- NOTE: this technique is over the vastus lateralis, rectus femoris, or vastus medialis, lifting the superficial tissue off the underlying musculature. Also, switching hands will switch the direction of the 'S' lift.

Muscle Rolling and Lifting Pectoralis Major

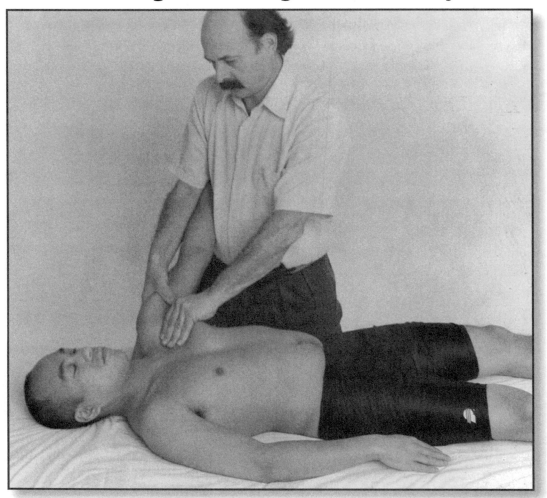

Performance Highlights

- The therapist stands in a low lunge position. Support the arm near the deltoid tuberosity with the outside hand. This hand will help lift and medially rotate the arm. Pincer compress the muscle with the inside hand. Both hands will simultaneously lift the muscle.

- Movement is created by using your legs, as well as your arms.

- Be sure that the hand that holds the pectoralis muscle is soft, using the flats of the pads. Avoid pinching or forcefully grasping the muscle.

- Respiratory effect: Both the client and therapist take in a breath as the therapist lifts the musculature toward the ceiling. During the client's exhalation, the therapist stays still, holding the client's arm and pectoralis muscle up off the table. Note that the client's body weight, as it drops toward the table, will create a fascial release.

Deep Forearm Lengthening on the Hamstrings

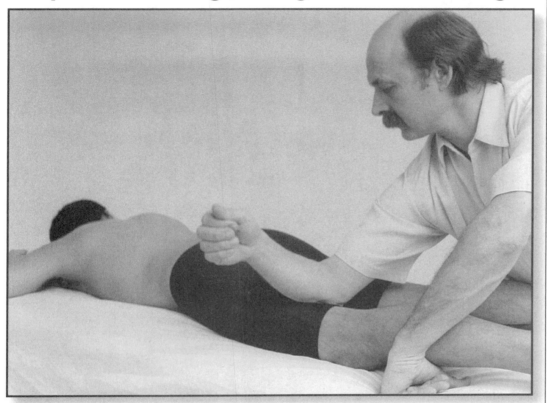

Performance Highlights

- The therapist stands in a low lunge position. Stand on the opposite side for semimembranosus and use your superior arm for the technique. Stand on the same side for semitendinosus and biceps femoris and use your inferior arm for the technique.

- Apply slow upward pressure toward the ischial tuberosity. You may try palmar or loose fist variations.

- You can be very specific to the hamstring muscles in this position. Perhaps try to integrate movement by asking the client to slowly lift and lower their foot off the table.

- CAUTION: Do not start your engagement near the popliteal region, or on the tendons of the hamstrings.

Forearm Elongation and Lengthening

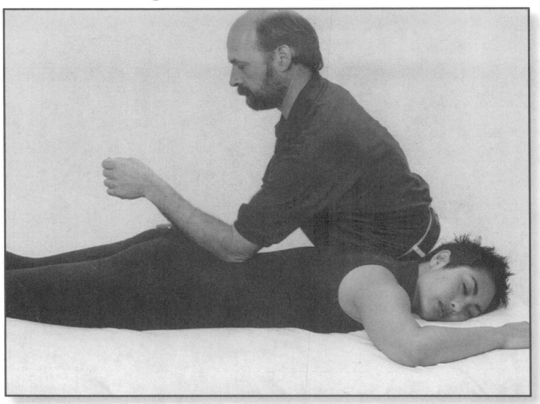

Performance Highlights

- The therapist stands in a low lunge position, facing toward the client's pelvis or head.
- Shift your body weight to change the tempo, direction, and to encourage the resistive areas to heat up and release.
- Be sure your contact is at the end of your forearm. You can change the intensity by raising or lowering your wrist.
- CAUTION: If you feel discomfort in the shoulder, try standing a little higher using your legs, or ask the client to move toward the edge of the table.

Pin and Mobilization of the Hip Joint

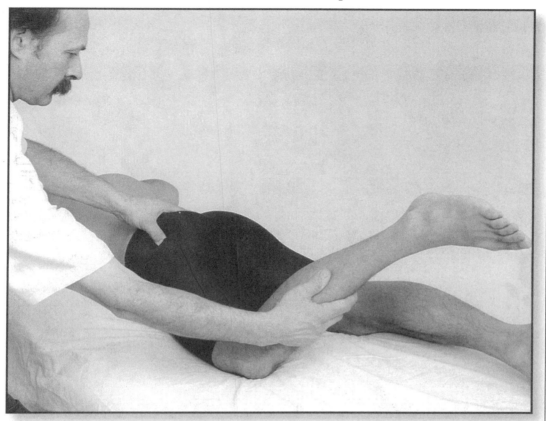

Performance Highlights

- The therapist stands in a low lunge position, facing the client's feet. Identify the top of the greater trochantor and locate the tendon of gluteus medius, then use your thumb of your superior hand for the technique. Use your inferior hand to hold the lower leg in a flexed knee position.

- Apply slow pressure into the gluteal tendon, while simultaneously moving the leg. Try medial and lateral rotations of the hip. Explore many combinations of movement while melting into the tendon fibers.

- You can be very specific to the gluteus medius, minimus, and piriformis tendons in this position.

Pin and Mobilization of the Achilles Tendon

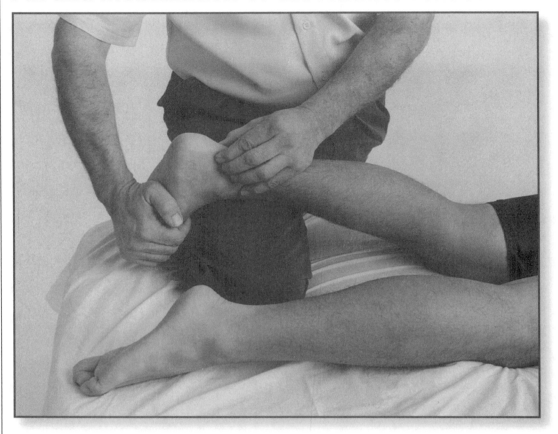

Performance Highlights

- The therapist stands at the side of the table with one leg kneeling on the table. Place the client's leg on yours and take hold of their foot with your inferior hand.

- Using your superior thumb and finger, apply a pincer compression to the Achilles tendon. Slowly dorsiflex the client's foot while maintaining the compression. This will create a gliding of the superficial tissue over top of the underlying calcaneal tendon.

- This can be very sensitive.

- Also add a variation of friction while moving the foot.

- The therapist can also perform this technique standing with the client's knee flexed to 90 degrees.

Pin and Mobilization of the ASIS Region

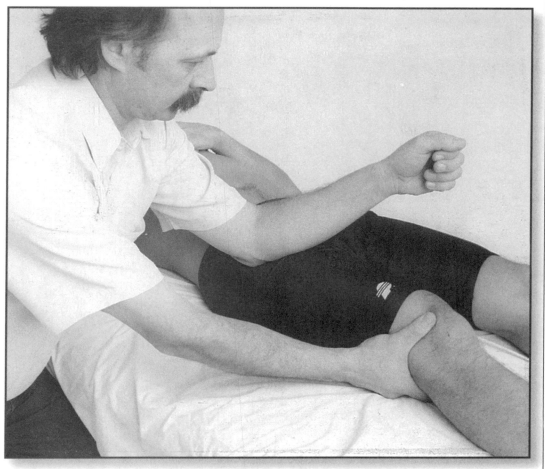

Performance Highlights

- The therapist stands facing the client's feet. Place your superior forearm just distal to the ASIS, with the hand pointing toward the opposite knee. Be in a proper lunge position, or kneeling position, using your body weight for leverage and angle of entry. Place your inferior hand under the client's knee.

- Be patient, using sustained pressure while simultaneously rotating the client's leg medially and laterally with your inferior hand.

- Ask your client to slowly rotate their own leg medially and laterally. This will help encourage the elongation of the hip flexor tendons: rectus femoris, tensor fascia latae, and sartorius.

Pin and Mobilization of the Wrist

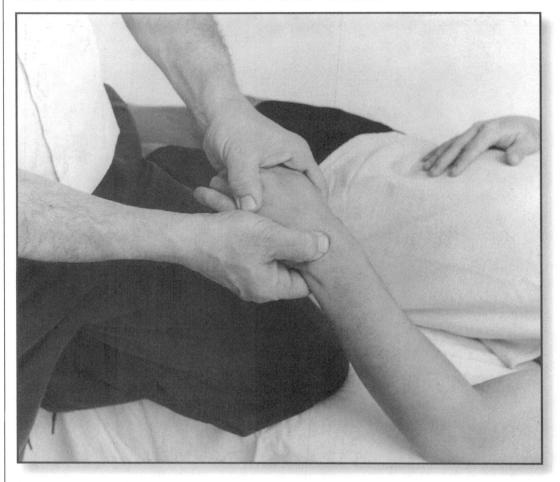

Performance Highlights

- The therapist faces toward the client's shoulder, holding the client's hand in one hand while applying slow thumb gliding strokes with the other.

- You may incorporate gentle flexion of the wrist while simultaneously gliding across the Extensor Retinaculum.

- Friction is an effective stroke, applying it in the same manner as the gliding variation.

POSTURAL ASSESSMENT OBSERVATION GUIDELINES

Medical History
- Injuries, traumas, illnesses, etc.
- Is there a relationship between the client's medical history and postural integrity?
- Emotional component observation; tone of voice, tenor of voice, fidgeting, etc.
- Behavioral component observation; holding breath, writing intake form, gait or seating positions.
- Take into account the different societal considerations, is behavior affecting function, or vice versa.
- Take into consideration whether pain causing the posture, or posture is causing the pain.

Notes:

Client Comfort
- Advise the client to wear comfortable clothing that allows for viewing the posture yet is within the client's comfort level (spandex, bike shorts, leotards, etc.).
- Have the client walk in place or bounce up and down with closed eyes periodically during the process; this will help to maintain natural, easy posture for more accurate reading. Any muscular holding patterns due to fascial constraints will be evident for a brief period after the movement, before the client consciously starts to adjust his position.
- Avoid verbal remarks in reference to assessment that might be heard and misinterpreted by the client.
- Direct the client to look at a fixed spot some distance away. This will prevent the client from inadvertently changing posture in response to the therapist's movements.

Notes:

Documenting Observations
- Be careful to avoid judgment or assessment in initial stages of observation.
- Observe behavior patterns from the start (i.e., how does the client fill out the intake form?).
- List structural landmark observations first (frontal planes, coronal planes).
- List observations prior to interpreting musculature and kinesiology.
- It's helpful to create your own shorthand; this aids you in quickly recording of observations.
- Be sure to start with the client's feet in the coronal plane—the only fixed point in standing posture.
- Notice stance patterns each time the client walks in place.
- Notice arm and shoulder patterns after the client swings his arms while walking in place.
- Having the client periodically walk in place will show particular movement patterns that may be noted by the therapist, i.e. pausing after movement, then turning a foot outwardly, or swinging one arm more than the other.

Notes:

Postural Assessment Anterior View

Structural Landmarks	Soft Tissue Considerations

Please note any discrepancies side to side/right vs. left

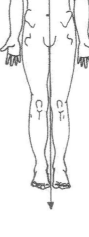

Mid-Sagittal Plane

nose (nasal septum)	rotation of chin and head
	(shape or thickness of Sternocleidomastoid)
manubrium of sternum	shape or collapse of chest
umbilicus	space between forearm and waist
pubic symphysis	tibial tuberosities in line with patella
equidistant between knees	(valgus/varus)
equidistant between feet	one foot planted more anteriorly

Transverse Plane

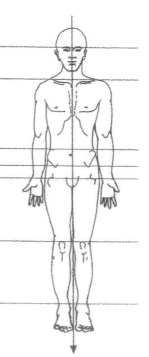

ears and eyes	asymmetry in shape of neck/shoulder
acromion processes	rotation of the clavicle
	rotation of humerus (elbow bent at 90°)
iliac crests	rotation of hands (knuckles showing)
ASIS (anterior superior iliac spine)	
greater trochanters:	rotation of hips (knee bent at 90°)
head of fibulae	rotation of knee/hip (foot rotated)
	top of patellas/asymmetry of patellas
medial malleoli	grasping with toes/bunions

Postural Assessment Lateral View

Structural Landmarks	Soft Tissue Considerations

Coronal/Frontal Plane

auditory meatus	shape of cervical curve
	shape of thoracic and lumbar curve
head of humerus	rotation of shoulder
	(humerus over trochanter)
	collapsed chest
	middle finger in line with iliotibial tract
	flexion of elbow
ASIS/PSIS relationship	anterior pelvic tilt
greater trochanter	texture/tightness of quadriceps
	texture/tightness of hamstrings
lateral epicondyle of femur	hyperextension of knees (or soft knees)
	one knee more anterior than the other
lateral malleolus (slightly anterior)	one foot planted more anteriorly

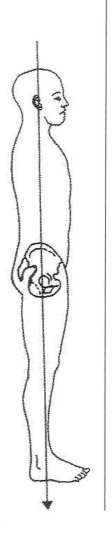

Postural Assessment Posterior View

Structural Landmarks **Soft Tissue Considerations**

Please note any discrepancies side to side/right vs. left

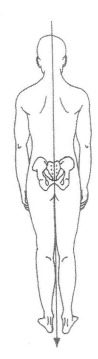

Mid-Sagittal Plane

Structural Landmarks	Soft Tissue Considerations
occipital protuberance (inion)	ears and occipital ridge
	cranial rotation/curve
spinous processes	equal distance between scapulas
	texture/thickness erector spinae
sacrum and coccyx	
equidistant between knees	equal shape of gluteals
	equal shape of calves
equidistant between feet	one foot planted more anteriorly

Transverse Plane

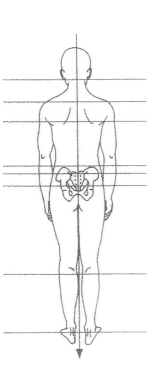

Structural Landmarks	Soft Tissue Considerations
acromion process	thickness of upper/middle trapezius
inferior angles of scapulae	rotation of scapula
	texture/muscular lines;
	(between scapula and spine)
	(between spine and ribs)
iliac crests	space between arms/waist
	lateral curve/shape difference at hips
PSIS	
greater trochanter	gluteal fold
	texture/muscular lines of hamstrings
head of fibulae	
medial malleoli	bow of Achilles tendon (arches)

UPPER QUARTER SYNDROME

Student objectives:

1. Define Upper Quarter Syndrome

2. Identify the postural distortions typical of Upper Quarter Syndrome

   - Forward head posture
   - Hyper-kyphosis
   - Three shoulder imbalance

3. Describe causal factors a client may present to the therapist (predisposing and perpetuating factors) that may lead to an Upper Quarter Postural Distortion

4. Perform assessment tests to identify features of Upper Quarter Syndrome

   - Postural assessment
   - Range of Motion (active and passive)
   - Shoulder abduction assessment
   - Neck flexion (chin poke) assessment

5. Design a treatment plan for a client with Upper Quarter Syndrome

6. Perform, demonstrate, and instruct a client in performing the Brugger Exercise and discuss its benefits

7. Discuss and instruct a client in self-care measures for Upper Quarter Syndrome

Upper Quarter Syndrome: A predictable pattern of dysfunction in which muscles of the upper quadrant that are typically tight form one component of the changes in the shoulder complex and axial skeletal systems and those that are typically weak form the other compensating component.

Muscular Involvement in Upper Quarter Syndrome

Features the following imbalance between muscles:

- Muscles—tightened and shortened
  - Pectorals, Rectus Abdominis, Sternocleidomastoid, Upper Trapezius
- Muscles—weakened and develop adhesions and fibrosis
  - Posterior Deltoid, Infraspinatus, Rhomboids, Serratus Anterior, Lower and Middle, Teres Minor, Trapezius

Three Individual Postural Components To Upper Quarter Syndrome

Forward Head Posture: Tightness and shortening of Sternocleidomastoid, Suboccipitals, Upper Trapezius, Semispinalis Capitis, Splenii Group

Hyper-Kyphosis: Forward collapse of the axial spine; tightness and shortening of upper Rectus Abdominis, weakness in thoracic Erector Spinae

Three Shoulder Imbalance: Tightness and shortening of medial rotators, protractors, elevators; weakness and elongation in lateral rotators, retractors, depressors

Postural Signs and Symptoms of Upper Quarter Syndrome

1. The occiput and top three cervical vertebrae will overextend, with the head translated forward, often in a chin-poking posture. This can lead to headaches, vision disturbance, jaw tightness, and compression of the atlas and axis.

2. The lower cervicals to the 4th thoracic vertebrae will be posturally stressed, often painful, and can lead to arthritic or disc problems. Due to the strain of compressive force, fascia may thicken in this region.

3. Elevation, protraction, and internal rotation occur at the shoulder girdle, generating neck, upper back, and shoulder muscular strain.

FORWARD HEAD POSTURE

In this chronic postural position, the head is anterior to the coronal plane. Two bony landmarks used to assess for this condition are the auditory meatus and the head of the humerus.

With forward head posture, the neck flexors are in a concentrically shortened position, giving rise to ischemia and hypertension. The muscles involved are sternocleidomastoid, scalenes, anterior neck muscles, platysma, and some hyoid muscles.

In addition, the neck extensor muscles in the lower cervical and upper thoracic region are held in an eccentrically strained position. This results in fascial thickening and fibrotic buildup, especially around the C6-T2 vertebrae. Many of these muscles are ischemic and have trigger points and myofascial pain. The muscles involved are the lower portion of Splenius Capitis and Cervicis, Trapezius II, Rhomboids, and lower portion Semispinalis Capitis.

Causal and Perpetuating Factors

Causal factors perpetuating this postural holding position include:

- Poor vision and improperly fitting eyeglasses

- Work and play conditions that require a slumped position or looking downward

- Gross trauma

- Posture reflecting poor self-esteem

- Seated positions

- Habits of bringing the head toward objects, as opposed to bringing the object toward the head (for example leaning forward to watch TV)

Vision and Postural Factors

- View obstructed by the lower rim of eyeglasses, which must be compensated by a forward tilt of the head in order to read.

- Having an undesirable posture with flat work on a low desk causing checkrein overload of the posterior cervical muscles. This may be aggravated by lenses with too short a focal length and rims obstructing the line of vision.

- Lack of armrest creates a drag or pulling down on upper trapezius muscles.

- Lack of lumbar support favors reversal of the normal lordotic curve.

- A low table increases flexion of the spine.

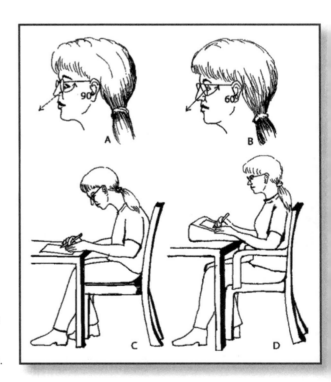

Car Or Sitting Posture as a Factor

A. Inadequate lumbar support; for example, sitting slumped in chairs or in most car seats results in loss of lumbar Lordosis, which causes collapse of the chest, forward rounding of the shoulders, and extension of the head in an anterior position.

B. Use of lumbar support corrects this situation.

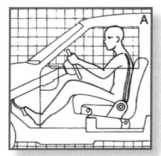 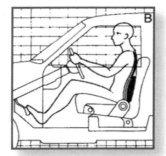

Three Essential Factors To Note Concerning Forward Head Posture Are:

1. For every inch the head moves anterior to the coronal plane, the implications for muscular and ligamentous imbalance or overload increase multiplicatively.

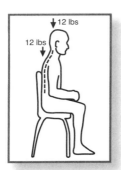 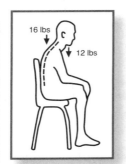 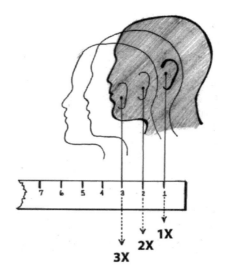

2. In the upper cervical and head region, both the flexors and the extensors are simultaneously shortened. The flexors pull the head forward and downward creating a downward field of vision. This activates the body's righting mechanism, requiring the head extensors to contract to bring the field of vision into a more normal horizontal plane.

3. If the person has no lumbar curve, they must be in forward head posture.

Forward head posture is almost always synergistically related to hyper-kyphosis. When one condition starts to develop, the other will naturally ensue.

HYPER-KYPHOSIS

In this chronic postural position, the axial spine is accentuated in the thoracic region. The upper portion of Rectus Abdominis is concentrically tight pulling downward, while the thoracic erector spinae are eccentrically strained and weakened.

THREE SHOULDER IMBALANCE

There is a symbiotic relationship between the neck and shoulder regions. The health of one is closely linked to the health of the other. "Forward head posture" is a common chronic postural distortion of the neck area, usually assessed by noting the position of the auditory meatus in relation to the head of the humerus. A closely associated condition found in the shoulder region is characterized by postural collapse. This postural distortion, often seen in combination with forward head posture and kyphosis, is characterized by three chronic postural changes in the shoulder girdle and gleno-humeral joint.

1. Elevation

2. Protraction

3. Medial rotation

The result of these three postural changes is a chronic change in the tonus of both the musculature per-forming these actions (the agonists) and their antagonists as well. Those muscles performing the action will be concentrically shortened while their antagonists will be eccentrically strained. Those muscles which are concentrically held will tend to be ischemic, matted, and adhered. Eccentrically strained muscles, overworked by constantly fighting gravity, will be weak, fascially thickened, fibrotic, dehydrated, and harbor ischemic trigger points.

Distortion/Action	Concentrically Short	Eccentrically Strained
Elevation	Levator Scapula Trapezius I	Trapezius III Serratus Anterior
Protraction	Pectoralis Major Pectoralis Minor	Rhomboids Trapezius II
Medial Rotation	Subscapularis Pectoralis Major Anterior Deltoid Lattissimus Dorsi Teres Major	Infraspinatus Teres Minor Posterior Deltoid

ASSESSMENTS

Supine Neck Flexion

Purpose: Assessing for weakness in deep cervical flexors and hypertonicity in sternocleidomastoid and suboccipitals.

Description: Instruct client to lift head and flex neck.

Positive test: Chin poking during initial lift off.

While the client is lying in supine position, ask them to lift their chin toward their chest. If the client initiates the movement by jutting the chin toward the ceiling, this may indicate overactivity of the sternocleidomastoid and suboccipital muscles.

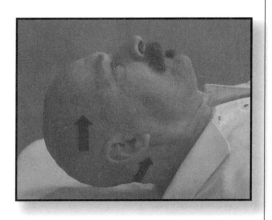

Shoulder Abduction

Purpose: Assess for compensating trapezius I and levator scapula.

Description: Instruct client to raise arm away from their body, while maintaining flexion at the elbow. Observe firing sequence.

Positive test: Hyperactive trapezius and levator scapula fires before deltoid.

Place the client in a seated position with his arm flexed at the elbow to 90 degrees and thumb facing upward. Ask him to raise his elbow outwardly. Note if the client initiates the abduction of the glenohumeral joint by any elevation of the scapula during the first 60 degrees of movement; if he does, this indicates an overactivity of Trapezius and Levator Scapula (neither of which should be involved with shoulder abduction).

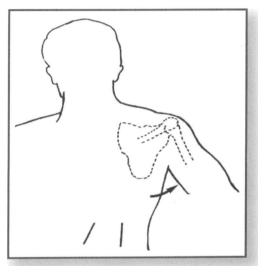

Janda 1983, Liebenson 1996

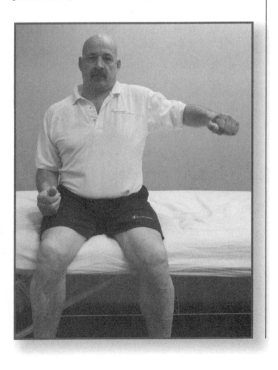

SELF-CARE MEASURES

Promote good posture by working with a higher table, a tilted work surface, a chair with armrests at appropriate height, and added thoracolumbar junction support to lift the sternum.

A higher table provides more adequate knee room, and the tilted board can be pulled even closer to the body for forearm support in the absence of adequate armrests. All of these contribute to a stress-free, balanced head position.

Three primary self-care measures the client can immediately include in daily activities:

1. Use of a lumber support while in a seated position

2. Brugger Relief Position

3. Self-Stretch for the Pectorals and Upper Rectus Abdominis

An additional self-care measure is the 'Wall Angel.'

BRUGGER RELIEF POSITION

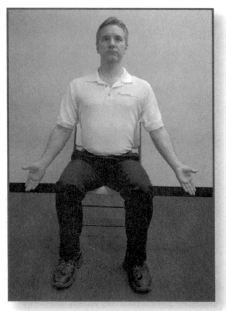

One of the most common causes of back and neck trouble is the sitting posture. When you sit, your body rounds forward, straining the joints, ligaments, and discs of your spine. Your muscles have to work as a checkrein against gravity and become tired and sore as a result. This posture also affects your breathing by compressing your diaphragm and encouraging excessive breathing from the shoulder and neck areas.

A simple exercise developed by a European neurologist has given relief to millions of sufferers. This only takes a few minutes a day and will improve your overall postural appearance within just a few weeks of practice.

Performing the Brugger Relief Position

1. Sit on the edge of your chair.

2. Place your feet directly under your knees and apart with toes pointed slightly outward.

3. Roll your pelvis slightly forward so that your back begins to arch.

4. Push your sternum forward and up.

5. Rotate your arms outward so that your palms face forwards. Separate your fingers as much as possible so that your thumbs face backwards a little.

6. Tuck your chin in slightly.

7. Holds this posture while you take a breath into your abdomen.

8. Repeat 2–3 times.

9. Perform this exercise 2–3 times per hour when sitting.

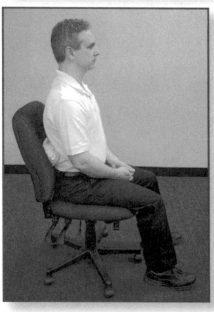

SELF-CARE EXERCISE:
STRENGTHENING—WALL ANGELS

Performing the Exercise

1. Stand facing away from an empty section of wall. Lean back, making contact with the wall. Stand with your heels six to eight inches from the baseboard, knees comfortably bent. Raise your arms above your head so that your elbows are bent and your hands are just touching the wall.

2. Perform a pelvic tilt so that your lower back is making contact with the wall (if possible).

3. Tuck your chin a little to lengthen the posterior cervical muscles.

4. Inhale. Then, keeping your wrists and elbows in contact with the wall, exhale and slowly lower your elbows to the level of your waistline (or as low as you can go without your wrists or elbows lifting from the wall). If necessary, consciously utilize muscular contraction to pull the elbows lower, keeping wrists and elbows in contact with the wall.

5. Pause briefly. Then, inhale as you slowly bring your arms back overhead to the starting position—all the time keeping your elbows and wrists in contact with the wall.

6. Repeat steps 4 and 5 up to 20 times or until you experience fatigue. This number can be increased as you become stronger and acquire more range of motion.

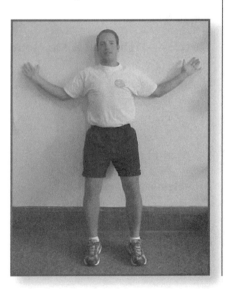

Special Instructions/Precautions

As always, if you experience pain or excess discomfort during the exercise, diminish the amount of muscle contraction or the range of movement. Perform the exercise slowly and be sure to consciously contract the external rotators and scapular retractors/depressors.

Frequency

This exercise can be performed daily.

Benefits

This movement reinforces retraction of the shoulder and neck muscles, stretching the upper trapezius, and stabilizing the shoulder through improved muscle balance. It is ideally suited for easing strain caused by forward head posture and rounded shoulders (protraction and elevation).

LOWER CROSS SYNDROME

Student Objectives

1. Define Lower Cross Syndrome.
2. Identify the postural distortions typical of Lower Cross Syndrome.
   - Anterior pelvic tilt
   - Hyperlordosis
   - Hyperextended knees
3. Describe causal factors a client may present to the therapist (predisposing and perpetuating factors) that may lead to a Lower Cross Syndrome.
4. Perform assessment tests to identify features of Lower Cross Syndrome.
   - Postural assessment
   - Range of motion (active and passive)
   - Hip extension assessment
   - Hip abduction assessment
   - Hip flexor length assessment
5. Design a treatment plan for a client with Lower Cross Syndrome.
6. Perform specific therapeutic techniques/stretches for Quadratus Lumborum, Tensor Fascia Latae, Rectus Femoris, and the Iliopsoas and discuss their benefits.
7. Discuss and instruct a client in self-care measures.
8. Perform, demonstrate, and instruct a client in performing core strengthening and stabilization exercises.

Lower Cross Syndrome: A predictable pattern of dysfunction in which muscles of the lower quadrant that are typically tight form one arm of the cross and those that are typically weak form the other. The Lower Cross Syndrome features the following imbalance between muscles:

Muscles—Tightened & Shortened

- Lumbar Erector Spinae
- Quadratus Lumborum
- Iliopsoas
- Rectus femoris
- Tensor Fascia Latae
- Adductors

Muscles—Weakened

- Rectus Abdominis
- Internal and External obliques
- Gluteus maximus
- Hamstrings

Short and tight: Lumbar back muscles

Weak and inhibited: Abdomin

Weak and inhibited: Gluteals and Hamstrings

Short and ti Hip flexors adductors

Postural Signs of Lower Cross Syndrome

1. Accentuated lumbar hyperlordosis, resulting in shortened and tight Multifidus, Lumbar Erectors, and Quadratus Lumborum.
2. Anterior pelvic tilt beyond five (5) degrees in men or ten (10) degrees in women, resulting in shortened and tight Iliacus, Psoas, Tensor Fascia Latae and Rectus Femoris; weakened and eccentrically strained hamstrings and gluteus maximus and posterior fibers of gluteus medius.
3. Overextended knees, resulting in strained Popliteus, Gasctrocnemius and ligamentous strain.
4. Compensatory hyperkyphosis and forward head posture may be present.

ANTERIOR PELVIC TILT

It is important for the student to remember that the pelvic girdle is a ball and socket joint, that is, the pelvic girdle is a component of the acetabulo-femoral joint. When a human stands and the acetabulo-femoral joint becomes weight-bearing, the femur becomes the origin (stationary) and the coxal bone becomes the insertion (moveable). This results in flexion of the hip, rotation of the pelvic girdle at the joint, and tilting sideways (abduction/adduction).

This allows the pelvis to be a very unstable region of the body, especially when the person is standing while being stationary or when walking/running/jumping.

Causal factors that lead to chronic hip flexion where the coxal bone is tilted forward and the femur is the stationary origin:

- Sitting for long periods. This leads to concentrically tight hip flexors.

- Sleep positions that lead to continuous flexion of the hip.

- Lack of use of hip extensors, particularly gluteus maximus, when rising from a seated position, lowering into a seated position, or when walking up stairs. Many people lean forward when rising from or lowering into seated positions, putting the axis point into the knee joint instead of the hip joint. This leads to atrophy of gluteus maximus. The same happens when going up stairs or steep inclines. This atrophy of the antagonist gluteus maximus allows for hypertonicity of the hip flexors.

It is important to know that when a person stands up after being in a hip flexed position for an extended period of time, the hypertonicity of Tensor Fascia Latae, Rectus Femoris and Iliopsoas will keep the person in hip flexion, and thus anterior pelvic tilt.

HYPERLORDOSIS

Hyperlordosis is often due to anterior pelvic tilt (tight hip flexors), when the person is vertical and standing the compensatory reaction is for the lumbar extensors to overly contract, pulling the person into a more upright position. This over-reaction is what creates the hyperlordosis. Thus, it could in many cases be that hyperlordosis is a secondary postural distortion to anterior pelvic tilt; that is, secondary postural distortion to overly tight and overly active hip flexors: thus, Lower Cross Syndrome.

OVEREXTENDED KNEES

When the weight is forward to the axis in the coronal plane, the result is the person locking their knees backward into full extension in order to gain more balance. This may result in one knee being more backward than the other. Also, the person may stand with one leg more forward than the other.

ASSESSMENTS

Hip Abduction

Purpose: To check for muscular firing sequence of hip abduction.

Description: With the client in side lying position, palpate the lumbar and gluteal regions. Instruct the client to raise the leg toward the ceiling while feeling the firing sequence of Gluteus Medius, Quadratus Lumborum. The ideal activation sequence if Gluteus Medius initiating the action before the lumbar region.

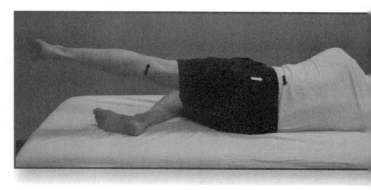

Positive test:

1. If the lumbar region "dips" in order to raise the leg, indicating an over active QL.

2. If the leg goes into a flexion of the hip, indicating an over active TFL

3. If the leg goes into a lateral rotation of the hip by turning the foot outwardly, indicating an over active piriformis.

Hip Extension

Purpose: To check for muscular firing sequence of hip extension.

Description: With the client prone, palpate the lumbar, gluteal and hamstring regions. Instruct the client to raise the leg toward the ceiling while feeling the firing sequence of Gluteus Maximus, hamstrings, and lumbar erectors. The ideal activation sequence is Gluteus Maximus and hamstrings, then lumbar erectors.

Positive test: If hamstrings or erectors fire first it indicates adaptive shortening. If the knee flexes it indicates an over active hamstring.

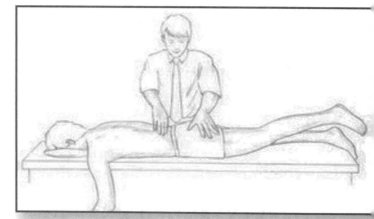

Janda 1983, Liebenson 1996

Hip Flexor Assessment

Purpose: To assess the length of Iliopsoas and rectus femoris.

Description: With back flat on the table, client should be able to bring the knee toward the chest to at least 90° without thigh lifting off of the table. In the same position, the knee should be able to flex to 80°.

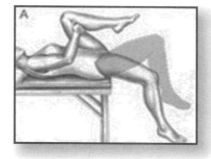
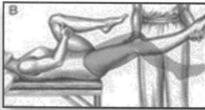

Travell and Simmons, 1983

Positive test: If the hip joint remains in flexion that indicates a shortened Iliopsoas. Knee extension indicates a shortened Rectus Femoris.

Self-Care Measures

Three primary self care measures the client can immediately include in their daily activities:

1. Self psoas stretches

2. Bridges for teaching the Gluteus Maximus to contract simultaneously with Rectus Abdominis

3. Pelvic Tilts

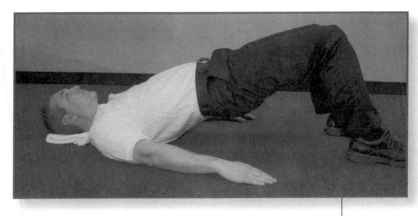

4. Self Rectus Femoris stretches, keeping the pelvis tucked

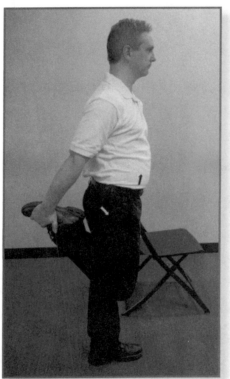

5. Positive Rest Position

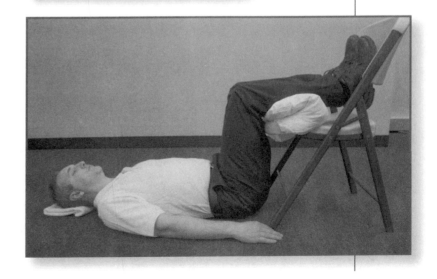